The
MRCPsych
Study
Manual

The MRCPsych Study Manual

Edited by Ben Green

Contributions by

Ben Green, MB, ChB, MRCPsych,
Lecturer in Psychological Medicine, Royal Liverpool University Hospital

Aideen O'Halloran, MB, ChB, MRCPsych, MRCP,
Senior Registrar in Psychiatry, Scott Clinic, Prescot, Merseyside

Paul Miller, MB, ChB, MRCPsych,
Lecturer in Psychological Medicine, Royal Liverpool University Hospital

Christina Routh, MB, ChB, MRCPsych,
Registrar in Child and Adolescent Psychiatry, Royal Liverpool Children's Hospital

Kenneth Wilson, MB, ChB, MPhil, MRCPsych,
Senior Lecturer in the Psychiatry of Old Age, University of Liverpool

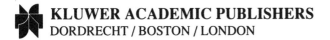
KLUWER ACADEMIC PUBLISHERS
DORDRECHT / BOSTON / LONDON

Please note that all case histories in the Patient Management Problems are fictitious and any resemblance to an actual person, living or dead, is purely coincidental.

Distributors

---

for the United States and Canada: Kluwer Academic Publishers, PO Box 358, Accord Station, Hingham, MA 02018-0358, USA
for all other countries: Kluwer Academic Publishers Group, Distribution Center, PO Box 322, 3300 AH Dordrecht, The Netherlands

A catalogue record for this book is available from the British Library.

ISBN 0-7923-8816-X

Published in the United Kingdom by Kluwer Academic Publishers, PO Box 55, Lancaster, UK.

Kluwer Academic Publishers BV incorporates the publishing programmes of D. Reidel, Martinus Nijhoff, Dr W. Junk and MTP Press.

Printed and bound in Great Britain by Cromwell Press, Melksham, Wiltshire.

Contents

Contents

Preface

This book is not intended as a text book. Nor is this book purely an examination aid. Its aim is to show the relevance of questions and subjects often addressed in the Membership of the Royal College of Psychiatrists (MRCPsych) examination. In showing the relevance of these questions and their relationship to current opinion we hope that candidates will gain a better understanding of the literature. Hopefully this will lead to a sense of how they can best organise their limited time for revision. Candidates can then gain as much enjoyment and knowledge as possible while they are preparing for their examinations. After all, the MRCPsych examination is not an end in itself; it is merely a symbol of a continuing educational process. We hope the book will stimulate the reader to work through its questions and through following up suggested references develop an expanding interest in the whole field of psychiatry. The ability to continually re-educate oneself will be a vital skill because continuing medical education will be a key feature in future European training.

The *Manual* covers both Part I and Part II of the MRCPsych examination, because the examinations are not discrete entities, but are parts of a training process.

The book should be used well before both exams. Suggestions for developing a study programme are given in the first section. The best self-study programmes will integrate time spent in ward rounds, case conferences, academic courses, 'self-help' groups and self-study. Notes on the most commonly-used reference books for MRCPsych are included.

The exam papers seek to give a guide to the level of difficulty of the actual examinations. The questions were designed to be as representative as possible. We hope that the exam papers can be used as tolerable practice exams under examination conditions and times. Practice in multiple choice question (MCQ) technique is vital in examinations where negative marking is to be used. Candidates often fear to lose marks by answering too many questions, when a simple truth is that unless they answer more than 90% or so of the questions they will simply fail to gain adequate marks. A breadth of reading is required for all the MCQ examinations. No single text is sufficient. Candidates in the Part II examinations are often surprised by the content of the MCQ examinations, particularly concerning the Basic Science paper. The choice of questions in the actual examination has been criticised for irrelevance by both trainees and trainers. Despite this, the general approach of the College is fair enough and some thought can usually prove the relevance of all the questions. That they often seem obscure or difficult is a reflection of the fact that the production of questions able to differentiate between highly selected and trained candidates is no easy task.

The MCQs are followed by answer sections which include true–false answers, often accompanied by extended explanations, with references. We have chosen the references carefully to cover many classic papers. Tracking them down and reading them will pay dividends.

Specifically for the Part II we have included an example short answer question (SAQ) paper, six patient management problems (PMPS), and a sample essay paper.

The clinical exam is the hurdle which brings down most candidates since a pass in this section is mandatory for both parts of the MRCPsych. There is no rigid, 'right' way to approach this part of the exam. However, there are classic pitfalls to avoid. Our section by Dr Wilson will help you to avoid them! A key element of success is to appear safe and conventional. No marks are awarded for radical heroism. An awareness of organic factors and a salient physical examination are held in high esteem, but will need to be counter-balanced by an adequate awareness of the psychological factors operating in your particular patient.

Finally, we have striven to exclude any errors, but as you will appreciate there is much detail in the book. We would be grateful for any constructive comments or suggestions that interested readers may make to help us improve future editions.

BG
1993

A Study Programme

Everybody studies in their own way, and so it is important that you design your own programme to optimise your chances of success. You will need to give consideration to acquiring both the knowledge and skills necessary to pass the MRCPsych, and since the exam seeks partly to establish whether you are acquiring the necessary skills to be a consultant, working for the exam complements your general training.

Although some people appear to relish leaving everything until the last moment, such 'binge-working' can lead to panic in the exam. In any event the gains in terms of study are rapidly lost after 'binge working' since the knowledge base is poorly rehearsed. The best method is to develop a programme where you can daily eat away at gaining the knowledge and skills required. The College has certain conditions it sets before trainees can sit its exams. The College stipulates minimum times that must be spent on approved psychiatric training schemes. Before candidates can sit MRCPsych Part I they must have spent one year training on such a scheme. The MRCPsych Part II candidate must have passed Part I and spent three years full-time in approved post-registration training. In addition, attendance at an academic course must be confirmed by the candidate's consultant and clinical tutor on his or her sponsorship forms. However, mere attendance at one of these academic courses does not automatically confer the ability to take the exam and pass. The course, like this study manual, will only work for you if you can put in additional time and energy: gathering knowledge through reading books and papers, attending case conferences/journal clubs, and seeing patients and formally presenting them (to exam standard).

The temptation to take the exam as soon as possible is understandable, but caution should be exercised. Extra experience is always valuable for the clinical part of the exam. Although an early pass (through taking the exam as soon as possible) can be advantageous in career terms, an early fail can be a blot on the CV (especially at the Part I level). Waiting at least until you are well-prepared will enhance morale when you eventually do take the exam.

Given the above arguments, you can see the desirability of starting your study programme as early as you can. Candidates for the Part I who read this book will presumably go on to be candidates for Part II, and so all the advice below is relevant in attaining your long-term goal. A short time set aside each day for this long-term goal will pay real dividends in your final revision.

What are suitable suggestions then?

1. You will need at least one large text for the exam. Since none of these is comprehensive you may need to find two. Unfortunately they are expensive, but they usually give a consistent and balanced overview which, hopefully, will accord with that of your examiners. Check with booksellers that you are buying the latest edition, or that a new edition is not about to appear in the next few weeks.

2. Think in terms of the exam while you work. For instance, if you are coming up for Part II when you are on a ward round or in clinic, analyse how your consultants manage their patients. All too often trainees adopt a 'cross-sectional' view of a patient. The immediate mental state is important, but a longitudinal view takes experience to evolve. Match your own ideas for management against senior trainees and consultants. Such a policy will make the PMPs easier.

3. View the group training activities in your hospital, such as journal clubs and case conferences, as more than imposed chores. Use what helpful feedback is given to you on your presentation, but don't be disheartened by any negative feedback. By rights all criticisms should be constructive, but sometimes in such case conference audiences there is an individual who enjoys looking superior. Test what they have to say, but don't let them destroy your confidence!

4. Start building up a library of useful classic papers that you have read or heard presented. You will need to organise these in some way so that you can use them efficiently in your revision. Depending upon how obsessional you are, you could distil the ideas that are most relevant and put them on a card index (or in a database if you are computer literate). The exam will probably not focus on individual papers, but on a body of knowledge. However, well-replicated studies may feature. Putting detailed references in your essay could be impressive if they are right and well-chosen, but they may be just irritating if they are wrong or spurious and will not enhance your paper. Read a few journals regularly. Review articles in the *British Journal of Psychiatry* and *Psychological Medicine* can be useful guides for further study.

5. Both at Part I and Part II levels, gather an informal group of colleagues who are all studying for the exam and organise yourselves to hear each others' case presentations and quiz each other on diagnosis (according to ICD-10 categories) and management issues. Not only will this give invaluable practice for the exam, but it will also produce a ready-made self-help group. The group needs to form at least several months before

the exam. To ensure that the group doesn't get into bad habits (e.g. all the group might be labouring under some misapprehension about exam technique), inject some outside ideas by inviting along a senior registrar or consultant to check presentation skills.

6. Either as an individual or as a group, try to gain access to a video camera to record your presentation. There may be things which you do completely inadvertently that seriously detract from the observer's confidence in you as a clinician. A slumped posture may convey an uncaring approach to the patient. Putting your hand in front of your mouth may affect what the examiners hear of your presentation. Lack of eye contact with the examiners may make you appear unduly schizoid! Video feedback can help you to change your presentation for the better and, as you see the positive effects of that change on subsequent tapes, your confidence will be boosted enormously.

7. Set aside a regular time each day for study and reviewing how your study programme is going. It is easy to ignore long-term goals while you are taking care of short-term demands on your time and energy. Before you know it, the opportunities for fulfilling your long-term goals have gone and only panic measures are left. The time you spend each day need not be excessive (you should aim to enjoy the time you spend studying, thereby reinforcing the behaviour), but it should be 'protected', i.e. without interruptions, and at a regular time, and when you are not too tired.

8. Although having attended an academic course is seen as an essential requirement for sitting Part I and Part II, it is a fact that courses in various regions differ and that your individual attitude to the course will also vary. Some courses set out with the explicit aim of getting you through to Membership, while others gear themselves towards generating skills and research. All these approaches are valid in that they will further your training, but you will need to adapt to the kind of course your region runs, profit by its strengths and rectify its weaknesses through your own endeavour. Try to interact with the course as far as you can. Look through the programme for the weeks ahead and consider adapting your individual study to complement it. Perhaps you could read the literature on operant and classical conditioning around the time that there is course teaching on the psychology of learning. Ask and answer questions during the course teaching – do not be afraid to make a mistake – you are checking whether you have understood the subject thoroughly.

9. Well in advance of the exam, write to the Royal College to obtain the most up-to-date details of the exam and available past papers. Over time,

the exam does change, and, hopefully, evolve. There is no 'syllabus' as such but there are clear guidelines for study in certain fields (see Table 1).

10. Ask colleagues which books they are currently using and what they think of them. Below are several suggestions with some comments of recommendation.

TEXTS

Hill P, Murray R, Thorley A (eds) (1986) Essentials of Postgraduate Psychiatry, 2nd Edn. London, Grune and Stratton.
(Almost informal in style, covers a lot of the basic themes that seem to recur in College Exams. Stronger on social and psychological issues than neuropsychiatry. Second edition now dated.)

Gelder M, Gath D, Mayou R (eds) (1989) The Oxford Textbook of Psychiatry, 2nd Edn. Oxford, Oxford University Press.
(Eminently readable, balanced text. Excellent for Part I.)

Kendell RE, Zealley AK (eds) (1988) Companion to Psychiatric Studies. 4th Edn. Edinburgh, Churchill Livingstone.
(Good all-round and in-depth cover of topics. Rather sober in style. Geared towards Part II.)

Weller M, Eysenck M (eds) (1992) The Scientific Basis of Psychiatry. 2nd Edn. London, Saunders.
(Essential for Basic Sciences MCQ paper of MRCPsych Part II).

Organic Psychiatry

The general texts above will need to be supplemented by a specialised text such as W A Lishman's *Organic Psychiatry*, 2nd Edn, Blackwell Scientific Publications. A new edition may be in the offing so check before you buy.

Diagnostic Classification

The tenth version of the International Classification of Diseases is mandatory reading for both parts of the exam. Until it was published in 1992, the most clearly defined diagnostic system in use was DSM-III-R. It will take some time for examiners to become accustomed to all the nuances of ICD-10.

However, ICD-10 will become the standard for the 1990s, and therefore you will need to acquire your own copy for frequent reference.

World Health Organisation (1992) The ICD-10 Classification of Mental and Behavioural Disorders. Clinical Descriptions and Diagnostic Guidelines. 10th Edn. Geneva, World Health Organisation.

American Psychiatric Association (1987) Diagnostic and Statistical Manual of Mental Disorders, Revised Edition.

Spitzer RL, et al. (1989) DSM-III-R Case Book. Washington, American Psychiatric Press.
(Excellent book with hundreds of case descriptions, followed by discussions of diagnostic issues and differential diagnoses. Interesting to read the cases and see whether you can figure out the correct diagnosis – therefore useful for Part I and Part II clinical exams and also PMPs. However, be well aware of any differences with respect to ICD-10.)

Psychopathology

For the Part I clinical exam, a thorough knowledge of psychopathology is essential. Some authors have calculated that 66% of the Part I MCQs are on descriptive psychopathology and 10% on dynamic psychpathology, (Cohen and O'Halloran, 1989 – *for full reference see Exam-oriented Texts below*). General text books like those above inevitably have a section on symptoms and signs, but for the purposes of the exam an investment in a specific text is worthwhile.

The most contemporary book has to be Professor Sims' *Symptoms in the Mind*, published by Bailliere Tindall. Accordingly it draws on new work, for example in the linguistic analysis of thought disorder. The classic text for some time though has been Fish's *Clinical Psychopathology*, which, although at times wordy and abstruse, has some real insights. Karl Jasper's *General Psychopathology* was published by Manchester University Press in 1963, and has sadly gone out of print, so that copies can only be viewed in libraries. This large book is fascinating to read, for its breadth and its philosophy as much as anything. References to Jasper's work have occurred in both parts of the MRCPsych examination.

In both clinical exams you will be observed interviewing a patient. The questions you ask patients obviously conditions their responses. The examiners will be interested in how well you interact with your patient. It is advisable to use standardised forms of questions such as those in the *Present State Examination* (Wing et al., 1984, 1987) or the *Geriatric Mental State Examination* (1976, 1988). *Psychiatric Examination in Clinical Practice* by Leff and Isaacs covers basic aspects of the psychiatric assessment, but candidates may need to supplement it with other reading on cognitive examination.

Copeland JRM, et al. (1976) A semi-structured clinical interview for the assessment of diagnosis and mental state in the elderly: the Geriatric Mental State Schedule. 1. Development and reliability. Psychol Med, 6, 439-49.

Copeland JRM, et al. (1988) The Geriatric Mental State and AGECAT diagnosis in community studies. Psychol Med, 8, 219-23.

Wing JK, Cooper JE, Sartorius N (1974) The Description of Psychiatric Symptoms: An Introduction Manual for the PSE and CATEGO System. Cambridge, Cambridge University Press.

Wing JK, et al. (1987). Further developments of the 'Present State Examination' and CATEGO system. Arch Psychiatr Neurol Sci, 22, 151-60.

Psychotherapy

PMPs and Essays often focus on the scientific basis for psychotherapy, and it is therefore wise to have a thorough knowledge of recent research (which can be accessed via databases and *Current Opinion*), as well as the more conventional outlooks and styles of various schools for which the following books might be useful.

Bloch S (1986) An Introduction to the Psychotherapies. Oxford, Oxford Medical Publications.

Hawton K, et al. (Editors) (1989) Cognitive Behaviour Therapy for Psychiatric Problems. Oxford, Oxford Medical Publications.
(Well-written and concise. Tells you all you need to know to be able to start cognitive therapy. Since cognitive therapy often appears rather mysterious it is pleasing to read such a helpful book. Useful if you are asked in PMPs, Essays or SAQs to explain stages in cognitive therapy.)

Malan DH (1979) Individual Psychotherapy and the Science of Psychodynamics. London, Butterworths.
(Comprehensible account of psychodynamic psychotherapy with clear case examples.)

Garfield SL, Bergin AE (1986) Handbook of Psychotherapy and Behavior Change. New York, John Wiley and Sons.
(Interesting and comprehensive account of psychotherapy research. Bear in mind that important research has been published since this third edition.)

Neurology

A good working knowledge of neurology, neurophysiology and the neuro-anatomy behind clinical examination is essential for both parts of the exam. No single text addresses all these needs and has up-to-date sections on, say, the impact of HIV as a disease entity or new methods of brain imaging.

Bannister R (1985) Brain's Clinical Neurology, 6th Edn. Oxford, Oxford University Press.

Barr ML, Kiernan JA (1988) The Human Nervous System, 5th Edn. Philadelphia, Lippincott.
(Current undergraduate text, but probably all that can be coped with!)

Carpenter RHS (1990) Neurophysiology, 2nd Edn. London, Edward Arnold.
(All you ever wished to know about neurophysiology and more.)

Draper IT (1985) Lecture Notes in Neurology. London, Blackwell.
(Basic, but well-written and comprehensible.)

Research Methods

Details of research methods feature in the Part II Basic Sciences MCQs. More extended descriptions of research and statistical methods regularly feature as essays and SAQs.

Freeman C, Tyrer P (eds) (1992) Research Methods in Psychiatry, 2nd Edn. London, Gaskell.
(The best text available in this field at Membership level. Comprehensive and interesting.)

Mental Health Act

Department of Health and Welsh Office (1990) Code of Practice. Mental Health Act 1983. London, HMSO.
(English and Welsh candidates may find the Code a useful resource. If you

introduce concepts from the Code into discussions in Patient Management Problems and Clinical Topics it will give the impression that you have a good and up-to-date working knowledge of the Act.)

Bluglass R (1984) A Guide to the Mental Health Act 1983. Edinburgh, Churchill Livingstone.
(Not totally user-friendly, but incorporates some useful points.)

Journals and Papers

Try reading the following journals regularly:

British Journal of Psychiatry
American Journal of Psychiatry
Acta Psychiatrica Scandinavica
Psychological Medicine
Current Opinion in Psychiatry
Biological Psychiatry

Obtain copies of the rather daunting *College Reading Lists* (published for various subject headings) and read at least some of the references.

The review articles in *Psychological Medicine* are worth spending a lot of time on. The Part II essay paper often reflects the general scope of these reviews.

Read *Health Trends* and the quality national press as well for articles on health care provision. Essays before now have used quotes from health ministers and editorials. The purpose of such informal study would not be to 'spot' questions, but to give you some general ammunition for such articles on debates in psychiatric care provision.

Management Issues

Elements of MRCPsych Part II may make reference to management issues and audit. Some knowledge of recent white papers, including *Working for Patients (1989), Caring for People (1989), and The Health of the Nation (1992)*, may be valuable. The *Psychiatric Bulletin* touches on issues of management with regard to psychiatry. A brief acquaintance with industrial management styles may be of interest, with regard to links between audit and quality control circles.

Bhugra D, Burns A (eds) (1992) Management Training for Psychiatrists. London, Gaskell.

Imai M (1986) Kaizen. The key to Japan's competitive success. New York, Random House.

Department of Health (1992) The Health of the Nation. Appendix C. Pages 81-91.

Exam-orientated Texts

There are many exam texts on the market, but we would only recommend a few. Exams often induce panic-buying close to the exam and unfortunately some books serve only to confuse. When you are close to the exam you certainly do not need to be confused. Books we would recommend include:

For Part I:

Bird J, Harrison G. Examination Notes in Psychiatry. Bristol, Wright.

Cohen RI, O'Halloran A (1989) MCQ Tutor: Psychiatry Today. Bristol, Heinemann.

For Part II:

Johnson BA (1991) Solving Conundrums in Clinical Psychiatry. Lancaster, Kluwer Academic Publishers.
(Useful for constructing ideas on how best to answer clinical management questions in the Clinical and Patient Management Problems.)

Hawton K, Cowen P (1990) Dilemmas and Difficulties in the Management of Psychiatric Patients. Oxford, Oxford University Press.
(Excellent book describing how to tackle such apparently insoluble problems as drug-resistant depression and neuroleptic-resistant schizophrenia.)

Psychology

A recent Royal College working party report, *Psychology for Psychiatrists* indicated how the College might put even greater emphasis on training in psychological knowledge and skills. Increased weight will be put on the candidate's psychological understanding of patients in the clinical exam. Unfortunately no single text currently addresses the needs of psychiatrists in training. To address all the areas in the current Royal College guidelines for psychology (see Table 1) will require you to read around the subject.

Gleitman H (1986) Psychology, 2nd Edn. New York, Norton.

McCarthy RA, Warrington EK (1990) Cognitive Neuropsychology. London, Academic Press.

Table 1: Areas of Psychology Covered in MRCPsych Part II.

Basic Psychology

Concepts of incubation and preparedness.

Social learning, particularly observational learning.

Sensory perception, perceptual organisation and interpretation set.

Information processing, attention and memory. Primary and secondary memory.

Factors affecting retention and recall. Chunking.

Cognitive processes and problem solving in health and in psychiatric disorder.

Theories of personality and how personality is assessed.

Extrinsic, intrinsic and integrated theories of motivation. Control systems. Self-actualization (Maslow).

Emotions: theories, e.g. cognitive, James-Lange, differentiation of emotion and development.

Vulnerability and invulnerability to stress. Learned helplessness and learned resourcefulness. Locus of control.

Arousal, consciousness, sleep, hypnosis.

Social Psychology

Attitudes and their influence on behaviours, stability of attitudes and attitude change.

Attitude questionnaires. How to communicate persuasively. Cognitive dissonance.

Inter-group hostility and different prejudices.

Interpersonal perception, attraction and friendship. Attribution theory. Dyadic interactions and social behaviour.

Leadership and social influence.

Small-group psychology.

Self-image, self-esteem, self-concept and recognition of self.

Aggression.

Psychological Assessment

Principles of measurement. Scaling. Norm and criterion referenced techniques.

Intelligence tests and what they measure. Definition of intelligence. IQ. Cultural influences and influences of mental illness.

Neuropsychological assessment and relevance to clinical practice in all patient groups.

Neuropsychological tests in detail.

Personality Assessment and Personality Function Assessment.

Sociology and social psychiatry

An elementary knowledge of sociology with regard to medicine is essential for Part II. Concepts such as stigma, institutionalisation, social class, race, culture, and sociological views on the family and society are bread-and-butter stuff and key reference papers should be thoroughly explored and essential details understood and memorised. The scope of the exam is reflected in Table 2.

Henderson A. An Introduction to Social Psychiatry. Oxford, Oxford Medical Publications.

Table 2: Areas of the social sciences covered by MRCPsych Part II.

Descriptive terms, such as social class, socio-economic status, and their relevance to psychiatric disorder and health care delivery.
The social roles of doctors. Sick role and illness behaviour.
Family life in relation to major mental illness (particularly the effects of high Expressed Emotion).
Social factors and specific mental health issues, particularly depression and schizophrenia. Life events and their subjective, contextual evaluation.
The sociology of residential institutions.
Basic principles of criminology and pathology.
Stigma and prejudice.
Ethnic minorities and mental health.
Methodology, particularly surveys, social anthropological and ethological approaches.
Inter-relationships between professional groups involving patient care. The characteristics of professions.

Child and Adolescent Psychiatry

Philip Barker's *Basic Child Psychiatry* (published by Blackwell) is a useful introductory text, but lacks sufficient depth, particularly in terms of research detail. The alternative is the comprehensive tome by Rutter and Hersov.

Rutter M, Hersov L (1985) Child and Adolescent Psychiatry: Modern Approaches. London, Blackwell.

BG

MCQs: How to Develop
a Coping Strategy

The Multiple Choice Question papers represent a considerable hurdle to most people taking the MRCPsych. Since the exam is taken by a highly selected group of people, who have already passed a plethora of difficult exams to become doctors, it is difficult to produce satisfactory questions that will differentiate between candidates. It is no surprise therefore to find that the questions focus on the minutiae. An MCQ statement such as *'Patients with Senile Dementia of the Alzheimer Type (SDAT) typically have cognitive functions which deteriorate in a sudden, stepwise manner'* might just discriminate between candidates at an undergraduate level, but not at postgraduate level where 100% of candidates will get the answer right.

It follows that it is essential to develop an eye for important detail and to read broadly, because the level of detail in the exam is necessarily high. In reading for the exam the candidate will have to negotiate territory that may at first seem alien to the clinical world he or she has been brought up in, particularly with regard to the Part II Basic Sciences paper. The Part I examination appears to be more relevant to the clinical world in that it does contain mainly questions on general and dynamic psychopathology.

Having read widely and wisely the candidate must then face the difficulties of negative marking and develop the necessary technique for answering an MCQ paper. Various books stress the importance of key words in the questions. Statements containing 'always' or 'never' are usually false. It is impossible to be so certain as to state that something never happens or alternatively always happens. The College MCQs are however of a high quality and would not depend on such blunt semantic cues for their discriminatory power. It is importat though to be clear in your own mind what the differences are between such important riders as 'pathognomonic', 'characteristic', 'frequent', 'often', 'usual', and 'typical'. The essence of a question may sometimes depend on such nuances. For instance, prosop-agnosia may be a recognised feature of severe SDAT, but it is not a characteristic feature.

Having taken on board the inescapable truth that it is impossible to succeed without learning enough and reading the questions carefully, we must address the problem of how many questions to answer. There are a variety of schools of thought. One is to only answer the questions you are absolutely certain about. This leads to a high proportion of correct answers, but runs the risk of not answering enough to pass. You may get 98% of those

21

you do answer correct but still only get 48% as a final overall mark. This is therefore a high-risk strategy. The second strategy is to answer all the questions, on the basis that, on the questions you are unsure about, you are still likely to obtain an overall positive score because you are making educated guesses. This is a medium risk strategy, because you may answer too high a proportion of the questions incorrectly and plunge into the abyss of failure. The middle-of-the-road strategy is to answer answer as many as you can of the questions confidently and then make reasonable guesses on a high proportion of the remainder. However, on those questions where you have no idea at all (to the extent that you don't even know what the question is about!), then perhaps caution is the best option. Questions which are truly unfathomable are perhaps best left out. However, a certain overall proportion of questions still needs to be answered anyway. A suggested level might be *at least* 85% (and probably more) of the question paper.

This where practice can help. You will have taken negatively marked exams before and used one or other of the above strategies at some time. You will know which works best for you. Practising your preferred technique on good quality practice exams can optimise your score.

In deciding your favourite strategy you might like to consider looking at the following MCQ.

The following terms are particularly associated with Carl Gustav Jung:

    A. word association tests
    B. Gestalt
    C. introversion
    D. the old man archetype
    E. character armour

Overall this question, when tested on a large group of Part I candidates, had a don't know index of 31% and a facility index of 0.49. However, different parts of the question were evidently easier than others. Answer E had a don't know index of 66% and answer C only 27%. Candidates were more likely to know that Jung was associated with introversion than the old man archetype and even less likely to know that he was connected with the development of word association tests. That he was not associated with Gestalt was fairly well appreciated, but the last response about character armour was left by most candidates.

The moral of this analysis is that within a question there are more obvious elements which can be quickly answered to achieve marks. Responses B, C and D can be easily answered with moderate knowledge levels and will achieve a passable level. This might generalise to other questions too giving a 60% score. Unfortunately other questions will appear more difficult to the individual and he or she will be unable to keep up this 60% result, necessitating educated guessing. For instance, our hypothetical candidate might think he or she has heard of Jung's work on word association and therefore feel that it may be worth a chance to answer this as well, perhaps then achieving an 80% score, and probably a clear pass.

Unfortunately there are only risk strategies. There is not a no-risk strategy. The solution for most of us lies in optimising our chances by wide reading, developing an eye for detail and a good MCQ technique developed through suitable practice.

BG

MCQ Paper One

1. Features of Wilson's disease (hepatolenticular degeneration) include:

A.   abnormally high caeruloplasmin levels
B.   decreased ability to concentrate on tasks
C.   irritability
D.   personality change
E.   'knifeblade' atrophy

2. Bereavement:

A.   does not increase mortality
B.   increases the use of alcohol and tobacco
C.   is associated with hallucinations
D.   may be facilitated by 'forced mourning'
E.   may produce 'morbid grief' as described by Lieberman (1978)

3. Tardive dyskinesia:

A.   is associated with frontal lobe psychological deficits
B.   is measured using the Abnormal Involuntary Movements Scale
C.   movements are inhibited by anxiety
D.   is attributed to irregularities within the basal ganglia
E.   movements are improved by drug holidays

4. Characteristic psychotic symptoms include:

A. pareidolia
B. eidetic images
C. hypnopompic hallucinations
D. ambivalence
E. passivity phenomena

5. Which of the following contributions to psychotherapy are correctly paired with their originator?

A. Paradoxical injunction and Frankl
B. Defence mechanisms and Reich
C. Depressive position and Hartmann
D. Transitional objects and Adler
E. Structural family therapy and Minuchin

6. Typical features of parietal lobe lesions include:

A. dyscalculia
B. disinhibition
C. visual hallucinations
D. anosmia
E. body image disturbance

7. Features associated with bulimia nervosa include:

A. parotid gland enlargement
B. disordered body image
C. family conflict
D. dental erosion
E. body weight less than 60% of normal

8. A good prognosis in schizophrenia is associated with:

A. structural brain abnormalities
B. low social class
C. sudden onset
D. good psychosexual functioning
E. the presence of neurological 'soft signs'

9. The Wernicke–Korsakoff syndrome is particularly associated with:

    A.   vitamin B_6 deficiency
    B.   damage to the occipital cortex
    C.   confabulation
    D.   a retrograde amnesia
    E.   damage to the mamillary bodies

10. Behaviour therapy:

    A.   is associated with the experimental work of Skinner
    B.   for severe depression lasts 30 hours on average
    C.   may involve functional analysis
    D.   may use a token economy
    E.   is used in guided mourning

11. Which of the following statements is/are correct?

    A.   The majority of suicide attempters eventually do kill themselves
    B.   Mothers in their first postnatal year are at the same risk of suicide as non-mothers of the same age
    C.   Suicide rates peak in the summer
    D.   Homicide rates peak on Friday nights
    E.   Eventual suicide is more common amongst people who have previously left a suicide note during previous suicide attempts

12. Causes of male erectile disorder (impotence) include:

    A.   hypothyroidism
    B.   multiple sclerosis
    C.   anxiety disorders
    D.   antidepressants
    E.   antihypertensives

13. Tourette's disorder (Gilles de la Tourette's syndrome):

A. affects more females than males
B. may involve loud grunts or barks
C. is associated with coprolalia
D. may involve motor tics
E. is best treated with carbamazepine

14. Neuropsychiatric complications of AIDS may include:

A. elation
B. encephalopathy
C. memory impairment
D. cerebral tuberculosis
E. cryptococcal meningitis

15. Recognised features of Alzheimer-type dementia include:

A. prosopagnosia
B. amyloid plaques
C. loss of cholinergic neurones
D. dyspraxia
E. selective loss of neurones in the striatum nigra

16. According to Anna Freud, neurotic defence mechanisms include:

A. sublimation
B. isolation
C. projection
D. turning against the self
E. mobilisation

17. Dissociative states include:

A. astasia–abasia
B. Ganser's syndrome
C. agenesis of the corpus callosum
D. multiple personality disorder
E. pseudoseizures

18. Long-term adverse effects of lithium, independent of serum concentration, include:

A.   tremor
B.   muscle fasciculation
C.   hypothyroidism
D.   diarrhoea
E.   ataxia

19. Bipolar affective disorder:

A.   was introduced as a term by Bleuler
B.   has its onset significantly earlier in males than females
C.   has been conclusively linked to chromosome 11
D.   may be treated prophylactically with carbamazepine
E.   has a higher incidence in socioeconomic class 5

20. Negative symptoms of schizophrenia include:

A.   blunting of affect
B.   delusions of reference
C.   formal thought disorder
D.   avolition
E.   similar features to those of Crow's Type 1 schizophrenia

21. Episodic anxiety:

A.   is associated with mitral stenosis
B.   usually remits completely within a year of diagnosis
C.   patients may self-medicate
D.   has a familial basis
E.   has been linked to abnormal blood flow in the right hippocampal area

22. Obsessive–compulsive disorder:

A.   according to Freud (1895) was an example of genital fixation
B.   has been linked to Tourette's syndrome
C.   can be effectively treated with clomipramine
D.   if severe, can be treated by limbic leucotomy
E.   is more frequent than anxiety disorder

23. The following neurotic and stress-related disorders are categories in ICD-10:

A.   agoraphobia
B.   post-traumatic stress disorder
C.   panic disorder
D.   depersonalisation–derealisation syndrome
E.   neurasthenia

24. Huntington's disease:

A.   is related to an abnormality of chromosome 5
B.   has incomplete penetrance in hereditary terms
C.   is associated with a large margin of error in pre-symptomatic testing
D.   usually presents in the third decade of life
E.   has an average duration of four to six years

25. ICD-10 categories of personality disorders include:

A.   schizotypal
B.   explosive
C.   anankastic
D.   psychopathic
E.   histrionic

26. First-rank symptoms of schizophrenia include:

A. second-person auditory hallucinations
B. a fear that the IRA will murder you
C. a hallucinatory voice commenting on one's thoughts and actions
D. the conviction that someone else is always moving one's limbs
E. hearing one's name called out upon waking

27. Features of temporal lobe epilepsy can include:

A. automatisms
B. memory impairment
C. autonomic symptoms
D. hallucinations
E. abdominal 'fluttering'

28. The following substances are recognised causes of hallucinations:

A. dothiepin
B. 'angel dust'
C. lysergic acid diethylamide
D. cocaine
E. diazepam

29. Dissocial personality disorder:

A. is associated with conduct disorder as a child
B. involves antisocial acts followed by genuine remorse
C. is associated with alcohol abuse
D. can be effectively treated with tricyclic antidepressants
E. may respond to a therapeutic community

30. Conversion disorders:

A. include hysterical paralysis
B. may involve aphonia
C. conform to a patient's concept of a disease rather than a medical concept
D. include transsexualism
E. may often eventually be attributable to organic pathology

31. Partially reversible causes of dementia include:

A. Wilson's disease
B. Huntington's chorea
C. B_{12} deficiency
D. hypothyroidism
E. Pick's disease

32. Chlorpromazine:

A. blocks prolactin production
B. is used in status epilepticus
C. can be regularly given by intramuscular and intravenous routes
D. produces postural hypotension
E. is an example of a piperazine phenothiazine

33. Features of frontal lobe dysfunction include:

A. poverty of thought
B. nominal aphasia
C. disinhibited behaviour
D. epilepsy
E. elevated mood

34. The defence mechanism of denial typically occurs in:

A. hysteria
B. grief reactions
C. schizo affective psychosis
D. murderers
E. dissociative fugue states

35. Examples of third-person auditory hallucinations include:

A. "a voice inside my head saying, he's useless"
B. "the voices outside say: now he's going mad and he's walking around the room"
C. "the voice says: go and jump. Jump now"
D. "I hear these voices in the loft arguing about whether I'm to be spared from the mouth of Hell"
E. "my wife and I often hear our next-door neighbours discussing us"

36. Patients with mental retardation:

A. are more likely to have epilepsy than people with a normal IQ
B. are less likely to have schizophrenia than people with a normal IQ
C. cannot be precisely diagnosed in the majority of cases
D. are most likely to come from social classes 1 and 2
E. are more likely to suffer physical abuse as children than children with a normal IQ

37. The thalamus:

A. includes the reticular nucleus
B. has no connection with visual pathways
C. receives no blood supply from the vertebral arteries
D. can be associated with hyperaesthesia if damaged
E. has no connection with spinal tracts

38. According to Sigmund Freud, dreams involve:

A. a latent content
B. condensation
C. displacement
D. dramatization
E. secondary elaboration

39. Therapeutic factors that Yalom found to be important in group psychotherapy include:

- A. projection
- B. cohesiveness
- C. universality
- D. altruism
- E. catharsis

40. The following are essential elements in the alcohol-dependence syndrome as described by Edwards and Gross (1976):

- A. memory blackouts
- B. a compulsion to drink
- C. peripheral neuropathy
- D. a stereotyped pattern of drinking
- E. relief drinking

41. Features of anorexia nervosa as described in ICD-10 include:

- A. weight loss to 25% below expected weight
- B. in males with anorexia there is a loss of sexual interest
- C. binge-eating
- D. body-image distortion
- E. a dread of being fat which is an overvalued idea

42. The following terms are particularly associated with Carl Gustav Jung:

- A. word association tests
- B. Gestalt
- C. introversion
- D. the old man archetype
- E. character armour

43. Examples of anti-epileptic drugs include:

A. selegiline
B. vigabatrin
C. lamotrigine
D. clobazam
E. buspirone

44. Temporal lobe dysfunction is associated with:

A. auditory agnosia
B. homonymous hemianopia
C. global amnesia
D. schizophreniform illness
E. Horner's syndrome

45. Patients taking reversible monoamine oxidase inhibitors should be told they must avoid the following foods:

A. broad beans
B. red wine
C. high-alcohol beers
D. cheddar cheese
E. avocados

46. Friedreich's ataxia:

A. usually presents in the fourth decade of life
B. mainly affects the anterior spinal tracts
C. is often associated with an expressive dysphasia
D. is inherited as a sex-linked recessive gene
E. is associated with nystagmus

47. Components of the limbic system include:

A. cingulate gyrus
B. fornix
C. amygdala
D. inferior colliculus
E. globus pallidus

48. Recognised adverse effects of clozapine include:

A. catalepsy
B. spike and wave discharges on EEG
C. akathisia
D. hyperprolactinaemia
E. urinary retention

49. Causes of neuropathy include:

A. leprosy
B. systemic lupus erythematosus
C. carpal tunnel syndrome
D. nicotinic acid deficiency
E. porphyria

50. According to Fish (1967), disorders of perception:

A. such as illusions are sensory distortions
B. such as dysmegalopsia are sensory distortions
C. such as functional hallucinations are triggered by a stimulus
D. include receptive dysphasia
E. include dissociative affect

MCQ Paper One

Answers

1. A = F, B = T, C = T, D = T, E = F.

Wilson's disease results from an abnormally low serum caeruloplasmin levels, and consequently high serum copper levels so that there is a resulting deposition of copper in the CNS and elsewhere. Copper deposition in the basal ganglia results in abnormal involuntary movements. Deposition in the eye causes brown Kayser–Fleischer rings to appear and deposition in the liver leads to hepatic cirrhosis. There is an associated personality change associated with a dementia-like process. CNS effects can sometimes be substantially reversed by treatment with penicillamine, a copper-chelating agent. Diagnosis is by measuring caeruloplasmin levels and testing urine collections for the excess urinary excretion of copper. Wilson's disease has an autosomal recessive inheritance. 'Knifeblade' atrophy is seen in Pick's disease.

2. A = F, B = T, C = F, D = T, E = T.

Klerman and Izen (1977) reviewed various studies and concluded that there was an increased mortality which peaked in the 2nd six months after bereavement. The bereaved use alcohol, tobacco and medication more (Clayton, 1982). Rees (1971) described *pseudohallucinations* of bereavement which are a feature of extreme affect and searching. Forced mourning may be used as a behavioural treatment to counter the almost phobic avoidance of persons, places or items associated with the deceased. Lieberman (1979) described three types of morbid grief characterised by phobic avoidance; denial or absence of grief and anger with others; and recurrent nightmares.

Clayton (1982) Bereavement. In Payket ES (ed), Handbook of Affective Disorders. London, Churchill Livingstone.
Klerman GL, Izen JE (1977) The effect of bereavement and grief on physical health and general well-being. Adv Psychosomat Med, 9, 63-104.
Lieberman S (1978) Nineteen cases of morbid grief. Br J Psychiatr, 132, 159-63.
Rees WD (1971) The hallucinations of widowhood. Br Med J, 4, 37-41.

3. A = T, B = T, C = F, D = T, E = F.
Tardive dyskinesia is associated with abnormalities on various psychological tests including paired associate learning tests, abstract reasoning tests, constructional praxis, memory functions and others (Brown et al., 1992). Despite the association the direction of causality is unclear. Cognitive deficits in schizophrenia are fronto-temporal in distribution. Abnormal involuntary movements in general are worsened by anxiety. Drug holidays (where medication is deliberately discontinued for a day or a week in the course of continuing maintenance treatment) have been shown to increase the incidence of tardive dyskinesia, in some studies (Jeste et al., 1979).

Brown KW, White T, Palmer D. (1992) Movement disorders and psychological tests of frontal lobe function in schizophrenic patients. Psychol Med, 22, 69-77.
Jeste DV, Potkin SG, Sinha S, et al. (1979) Tardive dyskinesia – reversible and persistent. Arch Gen Psychiatr, 36, 585-90.

4. A = F, B = F, C = F, D = F, E = T.
Passivity phenomena are Schneiderian first-rank symptoms. All the others can occur normally and commonly. Pareidolia is where ill-defined sense impressions (e.g. staring into the fire) conjure up ill-formed and fleeting images. Eidetic images are those brought into mind by memory, for instance the skill that some people have to visualise pages of a book once read. An exaggerated ambivalence was thought by Bleuler to be a distinguishing feature of schizophrenia, exemplified by ambitendence. However, a lesser ambivalence is part of everyday life for all of us. Hypnopompic and hypnagogic hallucinations occur on the threshold of sleep and are not indicative of psychotic illness.

Fish F (1967) Clinical Psychopathology. Bristol, Wright.

5. A = T, B = F, C = F, D = F, E = T.
Paradoxical injunctions concern advice to the patient to act in a way that at first may seem to risk making the problem worse. A classic injunction is in the psychosexual therapy of Masters and Johnson, (1970) where couples with sexual difficulties are told to avoid sex completely during the therapy. The prohibition serves only to heighten desire and re-inforce the sexual act. Other injunctions might involve prescribing symptoms, e.g. in patients with panic attacks, telling them to have four attacks a day (Frankl, 1970). Defence mechanisms were elaborated by Sigmund Freud and his daughter, Anna. The depressive position and the paranoid–schizoid position were described by

Melanie Klein (Klein, 1961). It was Donald Winnicott, a paediatrician and psychoanalyst who devised a pragmatic child psychotherapy and developed ideas like the 'squiggle game' and the transitional object (Winnicott, 1971), which added to object relations theory.

Frankl, VE (ed) (1970) Psychotherapy and Existentialism: Selected Papers on Logotherapy. New York, Souvenir Press.
Klein M (1961) The Psychoanalysis of Children. London, Hogarth Press for the Institute of Psychoanalysis.
Masters WH, Johnson VE (1970) Human Sexual Inadequacy. London, Churchill.
Winnicott DW (1971) Therapeutic Consultations in Child Psychiatry. New York, Basic.
Winnicott DW (1971) Playing and Reality. London, Tavistock.

6. A = T, B = F, C = F, D = F, E = T.

Typically lesions of the parietal lobe may cause: constructional and dressing apraxia, sensory inattention, topographical agnosias, prosopagnosia, astereognosis, cortical sensory loss, dyscalculia, dysgraphia, finger agnosia, and right–left disorientation amongst other symptoms and signs.

Lishman WA (1987) Organic Psychiatry. Oxford, Blackwell.

7. A = T, B = T, C = T, D = T, E = F.

In ICD-10, bulimia nervosa involves a preoccupation with food, bingeing on high-calorie food and attempts to mitigate the fattening effects of food by vomiting, purging, alternating periods of starvation, use of drugs such as diuretics and thyroxine, and a morbid dread of fatness. Bulimia may follow on from an episode of anorexia nervosa. Bulimia should be differentiated from upper gastrointestinal disorders (where the psychopathology is absent), personality disorder and depressive disorder.

Russell GFM (1979) Bulimia nervosa: an ominous variant of anorexia nervosa. Br J Psychiatr, 138, 164.

8. A = F, B = F, C = T, D = T, E = F.

Early onset, family history of schizophrenia, low social class, and IQ below 90 have all been cited as poor prognostic indicators in schizophrenia. Protective factors include marriage, female sex, and good premorbid personality functioning. Lack of insight, emotional withdrawal and blunting are bad prognostic signs (Wing, 1982).

Wing JK (1982) Course and prognosis in schizophrenia. In: Handbook of Psychiatry, Vol. 3. Cambridge, Cambridge University Press.

9. A = F, B = F, C = T, D = T, E = T.

Thiamine is the B vitamin implicated in the Wernicke–Korsakoff syndrome. The lesions in the acute (Wernicke's encephalopathy) stage can involve the walls of the 3rd ventricle, periaqueductal region, floor of the 4th ventricle, some thalamic nuclei, paraventricular nuclei, mamillary bodies, brain stem and parts of the cerebellum. Only rarely can lesions be seen in the cerebral cortex. Confabulation is a variable sign, usually in the acute stages. Other clinical features in the acute phase involve nystagmus, lateral rectus weakness, ataxia, peripheral neuropathy, signs of malnutrition, global disorientation and memory difficulties. Importantly, alcoholism is not the only cause of thiamine deficiency.

Lishman WA (1987) Organic Psychiatry. London, Blackwell.

10. A = T, B = F, C = T, D = T, E = T.

Behaviour therapy led from the work of Watson and Skinner. An average treatment course for depressive illness would be 12 hours, (Blackburn et al., 1981). A functional analysis would aim to define the problem and identify key variables, such as cues, triggers, antecedent events, consequences, and modifying factors including primary and secondary gain. Where avoidance is a part of the abnormal grief reaction, guided mourning using a kind of exposure (to distressing thoughts, images or places) is useful.

Blackburn IM, et al. (1981) The efficacy of cognitive therapy in depression: A treatment trial using cognitive therapy and pharmacotherapy, each alone and in combination. Br J Psychiatr, 139, 181-189.

11. A = F, B = F, C = F, D = T, E = T.

10-20% of suicide 'attempters' eventually go on to kill themselves (Ettlinger, 1964). The standardised mortality ratio (ratio of deaths observed to deaths expected from age-specific death rates) for suicide by women in the first postnatal year indicates that the rate of suicide is only one-sixth of the expected rate, leading to the conclusion that child concerns are an important protective factor even in a high-risk population (Appleby, 1991). Suicide notes amongst 'attempters' signal those at higher risk perhaps of eventual suicide (Dorpat and Ripley, 1967 and Tuckman and Youngman, 1968).

Appleby L (1991) Suicide during pregnancy and in the first postanatal year. Br Med J, 125, 355-73.
Appleby L (1992) Suicide in psychiatric patients: risk and prevention. Br J Psychiatr, 161, 749-58.

Dorpat T, Ripley H. (1967) The relationship between attempted suicide and committed suicide. Compr Psychiatr, 8, 74-9.

Ettlinger R (1964) Suicides in a group of patients who had previously attempted suicide. Acta Psychiatr Scand, 40, 363-78.

Tuckman J, Youngman W (1968) A scale for assessing suicide risk of attempted suicides. J Clin Psychol, 24, 17-19.

12. All true.

In recent decades psychogenic factors were thought to be responsible for up to 90% of erectile dysfunction in men, but more recent work has established that in urology clinics 78% of those attending for erectile dysfunction had some organic factors, although contributory psychological factors could be identified in a third of these. Vascular causes, such as venous leakage, account for 30% of cases and arterial occlusion 5%. Intrapenile injections of papaverine, α_1 adrenoceptor antagonists or prostaglandin E_1 are now common practice. 90% of men presenting with erectile dysfunction can be successfully treated to some degree.

Kirby RS, Carson C, Webster GD (1992) Impotence: Diagnosis and Management of Male Erectile Dysfunction. Oxford, Butterworth Heinemann.

13. A = F, B = T, C = T, D = T, E = F.

Gilles de la Tourette's syndrome affects more males than females and usually has its onset in the first decade of life. It usually involves multiple tics (rapid, repetitive, co-ordinated and stereotypic movements) which are accompanied by forced vocalisations which may be loud coughs, grunts, barks or obscene utterances (coprolalia). Tics and vocalisations are more pronounced under stress. The exact aetiology is unknown. A link with obsessive–compulsive behaviour seems likely. The treatment of choice is currently haloperidol.

14. All true.

Neuropsychiatric complications of AIDS are legion and include direct effects on nervous tissue and the effects of concurrent opportunistic infections. In terms of CNS infection some of the most common include fungal infections such as *Cryptococcus neoformans*, viral infections such as *cytomegalovirus* and bacterial infections such as *Mycobacterium tuberculosis*. *Cryptococcus neoformans* can cause a fungal meningitis. *Candida albicans* may cause multiple cerebral abscesses. *Mycobacterium tuberculosis* may cause multiple brain abscesses detectable on CT or NMR scans. The CSF will yield tubercle bacilli. *Cytomegalovirus* may cause progressive blindness due to retinitis. *Toxoplasma gondii* may create a space-occupying lesion. Tumours like non-Hodgkin's lymphoma may arise in the CNS. Dementia may arise from the direct effects of CMV, polyomaviruses such as the J virus and HIV itself. CMV and HIV may respond to ganciclovir and zidovudine. Adults do not bear the burden of CNS HIV complications alone. By the end of 1992 the World Health Organisation estimated that there were 600,000 cases of childhood AIDS. HIV infection itself in children may produce developmental delays or neuropsychological deficits through impaired brain growth, bilateral pyramidal tract signs and motor dysfunction.

Aylward EH, et al. (1992) Cognitive and motor development in infants at risk for human immunodeficiency virus. Am J Dis Child, 146, 218-22.
Department of Health. (1992) HIV and AIDS: The Issues. (*A useful teaching resource divided into specialty modules. The psychiatry module has a patient management problem to work through. Available in medical libraries.*)

15. A = T, B = T, C = T, D = T, E = F.

Prosopagnosia is the inability to recognise faces and is characteristic of parietal lobe dysfunction. Selective loss of dopaminergic neurones in the striatum nigra occurs in Parkinson's disease.

16. A = F, B = T, C = T, D = T, E = F.

Anna Freud listed nine 'neurotic' ego defence mechanisms: regression, repression, reaction-formation, isolation, undoing, projection, introjection, turning against the self, and reversal. She also listed a tenth, sublimation, which she felt was more characteristic of health than neurosis.

Freud A (1937) The Ego and the Mechanisms of Defence. London, Hogarth Press.

17. A = T, B = T, C = F, D = T, E = T.

Dissociative disorders, according to ICD-10, involve a partial or total loss of the integration between memories, identity, sensation and control of bodily movements. The extent of free will or conscious control is difficult to establish. Past labels include conversion disorders, conversion hysteria and psychogenic disorders. Dissociative disorders include, amongst others, dissociative amnesia, dissociative fugue, dissociative stupor, trance and possession states, dissociative convulsions, dissociative anaesthesia, Ganser's syndrome and multiple personality disorder.

World Health Organisation. (1992) The ICD-10 Classification of Mental and Behavioural Disorders. Clinical Descriptions and Diagnostic Guidelines. Geneva, WHO.

18. A = T, B = F, C = T, D = T, E = F.

Acute toxic effects of lithium include nausea, vomiting, diarrhoea, muscle weakness and fasciculation, disorientation, ataxia, dysarthria, convulsions, arrhythmias and renal impairment. Long-term effects, independent of the serum concentration, include thirst, polyuria, tremor, weight gain (partially due to water retention), diarrhoea, and hypothyroidism.

Aronson JK, Reynolds DJM (1992) Lithium. Br Med J, 305, 1273-6.

19. A = F, B = F, C = F, D = T, E = F.

The term bipolar affective disorder was introduced by Leonhard et al. (1962). The mean age of onset of bipolar affective disorder is 30 years, but there is wide variability. Studies have attempted to show a linkage to markers on chromosome 11 amongst sufferers of bipolar affective disorder in the North American Amish community (Egeland, 1987) but replication has not happened, and difficulties with the study's methodology have diminished early enthusiasm.

Bipolar affective disorder is not more common in socioeconomic class 5. If anything, bipolar affective disorder is thought to be more common in the higher socioeconomic classes (Weissman and Boyd, 1985).

Egeland JA, et al. (1987) Bipolar affective disorders linked to DNA markers on chromosome 11. Nature, 325, 783-7.
Leonhard K, Korff I, Schulz H (1962) Die temperamente und den familien der monopolaren und bipolaren phasishen psychosen. Psychiatr Neurol, 143, 416-34.
Weissman MM, Boyd JH (1985) Affective disorders: epidemiology. In: Kaplan, Sadock (eds), Comprehensive Textbook of Psychiatry, 4th Edn. Baltimore, Williams and Wilkins.

20. A = T, B = F, C = F, D = T, E = F.

Crow and his colleagues have subtyped schizophrenia into Type 1 and Type 2. Type 1 schizophrenia is said to have a sudden onset with mainly positive symptoms (Crow, 1985). However, the concept although appealing has been criticised for failing as a model to describe reality (Farmer et al., 1987). Liddle (1987) argued for a three-syndrome model rather than a two-type model. The three syndromes in his model are psychomotor poverty, disorganisation and reality distortion.

Crow TJ (1985) The two-syndrome concept: origins and current status. Schizophrenia Bull, 11, 471-85.

Farmer A, et al. (1987) Cerebral ventricular enlargement in schizophrenia: consistencies and contradictions. Br J Psychiatr, 150, 324-30.

Liddle PF (1987) The symptoms of chronic schizophrenia. Br J Psychiatr, 151, 145-51.

21. A = F, B = F, C = T, D = T, E = T.

Mitral valve prolapse has been reported in up to a third of patients with anxiety disorders, and there is an opinion that people with anxiety disorder develop prolapse because of the excess demands on their cardiovascular system due to anxiety. Episodic anxiety seems to have a familial basis: at least 17% of first-degree relatives of patients with panic disorder have the same illness. In contrast, 'control relatives' had rates below 2%. Positron emission tomography studies have shown an increase in blood flow in the right parahippocampal area (Reiman et al., 1986). In a study of neurotic illness in General Practice, only 24% of neurotic illness had improved over one year. 25% had a variable course and 25% a chronic course (Mann et al., 1981). It is therefore untrue to suggest that episodic anxiety *usually completely* remits within one year.

Crowe RR, et al. (1983) A family study of panic disorders. Arch Gen Psychiatr, 40, 1065-9.

Mann AH, Jenkins R, Belsey E (1981) The 12-month outcome of patients with neurotic illness in general practice. Psychol Med, 11, 535-50.

Reiman EM, et al. (1986) The application of positron emission tomography to the study of panic disorder. Am J Psychiatr. 143, 469.

22. A = F, B = T, C = T, D = T, E = F.

Freud's hypothesis (1895) was that obsessional personality represented a fixation at the anal stage of development, and that symptoms reflected repressed sexual or aggressive impulses. A link has been proposed between obsessional–compulsive disorder (OCD) and Tourette's, leading to speculation that there is a common underlying mechanism between involuntary vocal tics and intrusive thinking in these patients (Robertson, 1989). Further work has focused on the higher incidence of soft neurological signs in OCD (Hollander et al., 1990).

OCD has a lifetime prevalence of 2–3% and is less common than anxiety disorder. OCD can be treated with behavioural techniques, drugs such as clomipramine, and, in severe cases, psychosurgery such as limbic leucotomy.

Freud S (1895) Obsessions and phobias, their psychical mechanisms and their aetiology. In: Complete Psychological Works, standard edn. London, Hogarth Press.

Hollander E, Schiffman E, Cohen B, et al. (1990) Signs of central nervous dysfunction in obsessive compulsive disorder. Arch Gen Psychiatr, 47, 27-32.
Robertson MM (1989) The Gilles de la Tourette syndrome – the current status. Br J Psychiatr, 154, 147-169.

23. All true.

24. All false.

Huntington's disease has been localised to chromosome 4. It has complete penetrance in hereditary terms. Pre-symptomatic testing has a small margin of error (about 2%). It usually presents in the fifth decade of life. The duration of the illness is 13 to 16 years.

Lishman WA (1987) Organic Psychiatry, 2nd Edn. London, Blackwell.

25. A = F, B = F, C = T, D = F, E = T.

Schizotypal disorder is classified as a spectrum disorder within the schizophrenia category. The category 'emotionally unstable personality disorder' (impulsive or borderline types) has replaced the ICD-9 explosive category. Psychopathy does not appear, but is expressed in terms of the dissocial personality disorder.

26. A = F, B = F, C = T, D = T, E = F.

First-rank symptoms of schizophrenia include hearing one's thoughts spoken aloud, hallucinatory conversations about the patient, a running commentary on thoughts and actions, bodily hallucinations attributed to third parties, thought withdrawal, thought insertion and other influences on thought, thought broadcasting, delusional perception, and passivity phenomena. Second-rank features include catatonic behaviour, secondary delusions and hallucinations other than those described above.

Schneider K (1959) Clinical Psychopathology. New York, Grune and Stratton.

27. All true.

The commonest source of epileptic automatisms is the medial temporal lobe.

28. All true.

29. A=T, B=F, C=T, D=F, E=T.

Aggressive or antisocial conduct disorders of childhood are associated with a poor outcome, marital difficulties, poor work records and social relationships, alcoholism and crime.

Robins L (1966) Deviant Children Grown Up. Baltimore, Williams and Wilkins.
Robins LN, Rutter M. (1990) Straight and Devious Pathways from Childhood to Adulthood. Cambridge, Cambridge University Press.

30. A=T, B=T, C=T, D=F, E=T.

Conversion disorder is the DSM-III-R term for hysterical illness, which is expressed in ICD-10 as dissociative disorder. In dissociative anaesthesia, the areas of anaesthesia may often conform to the patient's notions of anatomy rather than the doctor's. There is a problem though with assuming no organic cause in this group of patients. Occult organic disease can often be a cause of such apparently 'hysterical' disorders in adults. In Slater's often-quoted study of 85 'hysterical' patients from a neurological hospital, at nine-year follow-up a third had had their 'hysterical' label replaced by an organic one, and, of the 12 patients who had died, three had died from an illness which had caused their 'hysterical' symptoms. Thirteen of the survivors had gone on to develop significant psychiatric disorder.

Slater E (1965) Diagnosis of hysteria. Br Med J, 1, 1395-9.

31. A=T, B=F, C=T, D=T, E=F.

The answer to question one in this section describes how Wilson's disease may be treated. Dementias attributable to folic acid and vitamin B_{12} deficiencies may both respond to reversal of the deficiency. Partial or total reversibility of dementia-like syndromes may be achieved when primary deficits in hypothyroidism, hyperparathyroidism, and hypoparathyroidism are reversed.

Lishman WA (1987) Organic Psychiatry, 2nd Edn. London, Blackwell.

32. A = F, B = F, C = F, D = T, E = F.

Chlorpromazine is a sedative antipsychotic agent. It acts by central dopamine blockade and may induce extrapyramidal side-effects and hyperprolactinaemia. In very rare circumstances, e.g. in intensive care, it may be given cautiously intravenously to achieve hypothermia; however its use i.v. is generally to be avoided because of its induction of fatal arrhythmias. Chlorpromazine is an aliphatic phenothiazine. Phenothiazines with a piperidine side-chain include thioridazine and those with a piperazine side-chain include trifluoperazine, fluphenazine and perchlorperazine. Butyrophenones include haloperidol, benperidol and droperidol. Dibenzodiazepines include loxapine and clozapine.

Ashton H (1987) Brain Systems, Disorders, and Psychotropic Drugs. Oxford, Oxford University Press.

33. A = T, B = F, C = T, D = T, E = T.

Slowing of thought and motor activity are said to be related to dorsolateral frontal lobe damage. Expressive dysphasia may occur if Broca's area (dominant premotor cortex) is affected. Epilepsy may be a phenomenon of frontal lobe dysfunction e.g. Jacksonian motor fits. Euphoria and facetious humour are related to orbitofrontal dysfunction.

34. A = T, B = T, C = F, D = F, E = T.

In denial, some painful experience, or some aspect or impulse of the self, is denied. Denial of painful perceptions or images is a manifestation of the pleasure principle according to Freud. Klein thought that denial of aspects of the self was often followed by splitting and projection.

Rycroft C (1968) A Critical Dictionary of Psychoanalysis. London, Nelson.

35. A = F, B = T, C = F, D = T, E = F.

36. A = T, B = F, C = F, D = F, E = T.

Corbett et al. (1975) found that a third of individuals with mental handicap had ever had an epileptic fit and in the year before the study one-fifth had had a fit. Corbett et al. also found they could make diagnoses in 85% of cases. Mental retardation is more common amongst lower social classes. This is suggested to be because preventive measures and schemes meet with less success for various reasons.

Corbett JA, Harris R, Robinson RG (1975) Epilepsy. In: Mental Retardation and Developmental Disabilities. New York, Brunner Mazel.

37. A = T, B = F, C = F, D = T, E = F.

The thalamus does contain a reticular nucleus, which is different to the reticular activating system. The reticular nucleus is a thin sheet of neurons on the lateral and ventral surface of the thalamus. The thalamus is connected to visual, auditory and somaesthetic pathways. The thalamus' blood supply derives partly from the internal carotid artery, but mainly from the posterior cerebral artery. The thalamus does have connections with spinal tracts: perhaps the best known reticular pathways include the lateral and anterior spinothalamic tracts.

38. All true.

The manifest content of a dream is that which is remembered and reported.The latent content involves the underlying memories, thoughts, fantasies and desires. The translation of the latent content into the manifest content is the dream work. Condensation, displacement, dramatization and secondary elaboration are parts of that dream work. In condensation ideas are merged, so that figures in dreams may be composite or words in dreams condensed to neologisms. The condensation may act as a decoy to divert the dreamer from more dangerous themes. Dramatisation is the translation of thoughts into imagery and this is usually concrete in nature. Secondary elaboration refers to the mutation of the dream after waking, often by omission or forgetting.

Freud S (1900) The Interpretation of Dreams. In: Strachey J (ed), Complete Psychological Works, Vol V. London, Hogarth Press.

39. A = F, B = T, C = T, D = T, E = T.

Highly cohesive groups have a better record of attendance, punctuality, activity by their members and stability (Yalom, 1975). Universality enables patients to see that other group members have similar experiences, difficulties and feelings to their own. Catharsis must be linked with insight to be helpful. Yalom (1977) suggested that catharsis without an opportunity to integrate the emotional experience can have harmful effects.

Yalom ID (1975) The Theory and Practice of Group Psychotherapy. New York, Basic Books.
Yalom ID, et al. (1977) The impact of a weekend group experience on individual therapy.

40. A = F, B = T, C = F, D = T, E = T.

Edwards and Gross (1976) described the alcohol dependence syndrome which comprised a stereotyped pattern of drinking, prominence of alcohol-seeking behaviour, increased alcohol tolerance, repeated withdrawal symptoms, relief or avoidance of withdrawal by further drinking, a subjective awareness of a compulsion to drink, and relapse or re-instatement of drinking behaviour after abstinence.

Edwards G, Gross MM (1976) Alcohol dependence: provisional description of a clinical syndrome. Br Med J, 1, 1058.

41. A = F, B = T, C = F, D = T, E = T.

Features of anorexia nervosa as described in ICD-10 include body weight at least 15% below that expected or Quetelet's body-mass index is 17.5 or less. Quetelet's body-mass index is the weight in kilograms divided by the square of the height in metres. Other features include a dread of fatness amounting to an overvalued idea, body-image distortion, self-induced weight loss, vomiting, purging, excessive exercise, use of appetite suppressants or diuretics, amenorrhoea in women and loss of sexual interest/potency in men, raised growth hormone and cortisol, changes in thyroid hormone metabolism and abnormal insulin secretion.

42. A = T, B = F, C = T, D = T, E = F.

Jung wrote some of the earliest papers on word association. Gestalt is associated with the therapy style of Fritz Perls. Introversion and extraversion are personality types associated with Jung's work. Jung also suggested that there was a series of archetypes which were integral to all human experience and memory including the mother archetype, the old man archetype, the trickster and others. Character armour is a term derived from the work of Wilhelm Reich. He saw character armour as a persistent interpersonal defence mechanism. One of his examples was a female 'hysteric' who was continually provocative and seductive. Reich saw this as a defense to expose males whom she could not trust, for once the male responded to her 'character armour' she would spurn him. In this way, Reich thought, she could flush out dangerous males before they could damage her.

Jung CG (1963) Memories, Dreams and Reflections. London, Routledge and Kegan Paul.
Reich W (1949) Character Analysis. New York, Farrar, Straus, and Young.
Rycroft C (1969) Wilhelm Reich. New York, Viking Press.
Storr A (1983) Jung: Selected Writings. London, Fontana.

43. A=F, B=T, C=T, D=T, E=F.

Selegiline is useful in severe Parkinson's disease or symptomatic parkinsonism, but is not used for extrapyramidal side-effects. Selegiline is usually used in conjunction with levodopa and as a MAO-B inhibitor therefore reduces end-of-dose deterioration. Vigabatrin and lomotrigine are relative newcomers to anti-epileptic therapy. Vigabatrin may exacerbate or induce psychoses. Clobazam is an adjunctive treatment in epilepsy. Buspirone is an anxiolytic with no anti-epileptic activity.

44. A=T, B=T, C=T, D=T, E=F.

45. All false.

Foods such as cheese, which contain high levels of tyramine, are usually excluded from the diet of patients taking irreversible monoamine oxidase inhibitors such as phenelzine and tranylcypromine. Reversible MAO inhibitors like moclobemide, which are selective for MAO-A and -B, should eliminate the risk of hypertension through exposure to certain foods. They can be prescribed without any foods being eliminated from the diet, although a diet which was *exclusively* of large amounts of certain foods like cheese and broad bean pods might still be problematic.

Priest RG (ed) (1989) Depression and reversible monoamine oxidase inhibitors – new perspectives. Br J Psychiatr, Suppl. 6.

46. A = F, B = F, C = F, D = F, E = T.

Friedreich's ataxia has an early onset, between 5 and 15 years. The ataxia is secondary to a degeneration of the posterior columns, lateral columns, especially the corticospinal and posterior spinocerebellar tracts. The heart muscle becomes thickened and fibrosed leading to death in the fifth decade of life from cardiac failure. Recognised features include ataxia, upper limb in-coordination, nystagmus, intention tremor, dysarthria, nystagmus, extensor plantar reflexes, poor proprioception, pes cavus, scoliosus, and optic atrophy.

47. A = T, B = T, C = T, D = F, E = F.

The limbic system regulates the hypothalamus and is important for emotional and affective functions. The limbic system is also involved in the control of motivation and actions. It incorporates the olfactory bulbs and lobes, hippocampus, amygdala, cingulate cortex, the septal area, fornix, hippocampus and parahippocampal gyrus.

48. A = F, B = T, C = T, D = F, E = T.

Clozapine is an atypical antipsychotic and does not induce catalepsy. Clozapine may precipitate epileptic seizures by lowering epileptic thresholds in a dose-dependent manner. Akathisia, tremor and rigidity are adverse extrapyramidal effects of clozapine. High prolactin levels have not been associated with clozapine. Urinary incontinence and retention are both side-effects.

49. All true.

Leprosy produces direct effects on the nerve, causing neuropathy and thickening of the nerve with depigmentation of the skin. Nicotinic acid deficiency causes diarrhoea, polyneuropathy, glossitis, a dark, scaly dermatitis and sometimes a mild dementia.

50. A = F, B = T, C = T, D = F, E = F.

Illusions according to Fish are sensory deceptions. Dysmegalopsia and micropsia are sensory distortions. Dysmegalopsia involves a change in spatial form, and may occur in retinal disease, disorders of accommodation, and temporal lobe lesions. Fish's example of a functional hallucination involves a patient with schizophrenia who heard the voice of God talking to her in time with a ticking clock. Receptive aphasias are classified by Fish as speech disorders, and dissociative affect is classed as a disorder of the experience of self.

Fish F (1967) Clinical Psychopathology. Bristol, Wright.

BG

MCQ Paper Two

Sciences Basic to Psychiatry (MRCPsych Part II)
One-and-a-half hours
50 questions

1. In testing disturbances of information processing:

A.   the Continuous Performance Test (CPT) involves the presentation of target stimuli amongst random stimuli on a computer screen

B.   short-term recall memory deficits occur in schizophrenia

C.   a pendulum can be used to test smooth pursuit eye movement

D.   there is no relationship between smooth pursuit eye movement dysfunction and *chronic* schizophrenia

E.   the Wisconsin Card Sorting Test measures temporal lobe dysfunction

2. Personal Construct Theory:

A.   emphasises man as a historian

B.   suggests that personality is the sum of a cluster of neurotic complexes

C.   incorporates theories on creativity

D.   led to the development of the repertory grid

E.   suggests that people may sacrifice themselves to preserve core constructs

3. The Bedford College method of assessing Life-Events:

A.   allows both idiographic and nomothetic information to be combined

B.   rates life-events on a severity scale of 1 to 100

C.   rates events independently of their context

D.   takes into account how the individual *felt* about the event

E.   is a self-rating questionnaire

4. Sleep:

A.   during the night is mainly composed of REM sleep
B.   which includes most dreams is called orthodox sleep
C.   deprivation may lead to hallucinosis
D.   disorders may be associated with HLA DR2
E.   is associated with a reduction in serum growth hormone levels

5. Brain lesions:

A.   in the posterior right hemisphere are associated with prosopagnosia
B.   only cause constructional apraxia when they are in the right parietal lobe
C.   in the temporal lobe may cause jargon aphasia
D.   which cause any auditory short-term memory impairment affect visual short-term memory too
E.   which produce lexical agraphia are usually in the parietal lobe

6. Features of a good diagnostic taxonomy include:

A.   interdiagnoser reliability
B.   internal consistency
C.   specificity
D.   meshing
E.   external validity

7. Which of the following statements are true or false?

A.   The central tendency is another term for the standard deviation
B.   A t-test measures statistical significance of the distance between the means of two sets of scores
C.   A nominal measure has categories that are ranked, but not in terms of equal size.
D.   The probability that a given result could be caused by sampling error is called the Z-score
E.   The correlation measures the strength of association between two interval variables

8. The Parental Bonding Instrument:

A. is based on a 2-hour interview
B. measures dependency
C. yields abnormal care scores from neurotic depressives
D. yields normal control scores from neurotic depressives
E. measures bonding from the parents' point-of-view

9. Organic amnesia:

A. prevents learning through simple classical conditioning
B. · may be caused by lesions of the midline diencephalon
C. caused by hippocampal lesions is of severe anterograde and severe retrograde types
D. may be tested using the Boston Remote Memory Test
E. in Wernicke–Korsakoff syndrome is often anterograde and retrograde

10. Which of the following statements about the genetics of psychiatry are true or false?

A. Prader–Willi syndrome is associated with an abnormal chromosome 11
B. In Huntington's disease the age of onset is much earlier if it is inherited from the mother
C. Inherited maternal and paternal chromosomes function differently in cerebellar ataxia
D. 20% of males inheriting a fragile-X chromosome are asymptomatic
E. Sub-types of schizophrenia have been consistently linked to chromosome 5

11. In interpreting epidemiological study associations:

A.   a type 2 error occurs where there is no true association, but the *p* value is significant

B.   confidence intervals can be used to display the possibility of type 2 errors

C.   the association between schizophrenia and low social class may be an example of reverse causality

D.   spurious associations may be caused by a confounder

E.   multivariate analyses are only suitable for very large, community-based studies

12. With regard to perception and attention:

A.   perception at the absolute threshold is the highest intensity of a stimulus that can be tolerated

B.   dichotic listening can investigate selective attention

C.   the Stroop effect concerns rapid eye movement

D.   image processing beyond the primary visual cortex is usually serial processing

E.   top-down processing involves reading *down* the page

13. In genetics:

A.   the standard notation for gene location uses the term 'p' to indicate the long arm of the chromosome

B.   recombinant DNA is produced when plasmids are inserted into human DNA

C.   DNA polymerase chain reactions can amplify specific DNA fragments

D.   a criterion for significant genetic linkage is a lod score of less than 3

E.   the lod score is very sensitive to errors in diagnosis

14. In the use of psychiatric rating scales:

A. validity is a measure of a scale's ability to produce consistent results

B. concurrent validity is a comparison of test scores and suitable standard criteria

C. the Brief Psychiatric Rating Scale can measure change during clinical trials

D. the inter-rater reliability for the Hamilton Rating Scale is acknowledged to be low

E. average rating scales achieve inter-rater reliability scores of approximately 0.9

15. In expressing judgements about visual measurements:

A. an individual will usually change their decision if the group they are in expresses a contrary opinion

B. a unanimous group of 20 is much more likely than a unanimous group of 3 to persuade an individual to change his or her decision

C. an individual is far less likely to yield to a group decision if just one other individual agrees with him or her

D. the majority of individuals will stick to their own opinion in the face of group opposition

E. an individual can easily persuade a group to change their group opinion

16. In behavioural psychology:

A. a coverant behaviour is a covert operant behaviour

B. Skinner's theories only describe observable non-verbal behaviours

C. the concept of *shaping* is associated with J B Watson

D. successive approximations can be used to teach procedures

E. a response is much harder to extinguish if it was acquired during continuous rather than partial re-inforcement

17. In terms of British social attitudes:

A.   support for universally provided National Health services is highest amongst social class V

B.   most people feel that the quality of medical treatment in hospitals needs improvement

C.   more people are satisfied with their General Practitioner than hospital outpatient services

D.   there has been an increase in the percentage of people who think that homosexual relationships are 'always or mostly wrong'

E.   most people believe that in terms of judgements about fraud right and wrong are absolutes

18. Piaget was associated with developing the following concepts regarding the developing mind:

A.   the stage of formal operations

B.   object constancy

C.   conservation of energy

D.   genetic epistemology

E.   two-factor theory of intelligence

19. In terms of social class:

A.   the Registrar-General's classification has 30 occupational unit groups

B.   categories can be classified into Goldthorpe's schema

C.   the Registrar-General's classification is according to the current or last occupation

D.   the unemployed are automatically given an average classification of III non-manual

E.   senile dementia of the Alzheimer type has been found to be more prevalent in class V

20. In schizophrenia:

A. studies on homovanillic acid have demonstrated incrased dopamine turnover
B. the activity of tyrosine hydroxylase is raised
C. prolonged neuroleptic administration has been shown to be linked to an increase in striatal D2 receptors
D. D2 receptors stimulate adenylate cyclase activity
E. haloperidol stimulates brain dopamine turnover

21. In measuring morbidity:

A. the incidence rate is the number of completed episodes of illness in a year
B. the average duration of sickness is the incidence rate divided by the point prevalence
C. the point prevalence rate is the number of illnesses at any time over the number of people exposed to risk in a period
D. incidence is best studied using a cross-sectional survey
E. a crude rate relates to particular sections of the population

22. Parametric statistical methods:

A. usually rely on ranking procedures
B. do not include Student's t distribution
C. are usually used after non-parametric methods have been tried
D. include the Chi-squared distribution
E. depend on assumptions about distribution

23. Reasonably consistent findings in recent epidemiological studies have demonstrated that:

A. head injury is associated with later idiopathic dementia
B. heavy alcohol consumption is associated with later dementia
C. elderly depressive are more likely than younger depressives to have a family history of affective disorders
D. prevalence rates for schizophrenia are stable across temporal and geographical boundaries
E. women with schizophrenia tend to have more affective symptoms than men

24. In assessing personality:

A.   the Minnesota Multiphasic Personality Inventory has a
      schizophrenia scale
B.   the California Personality Inventory was developed for a
      psychiatric population
C.   the Thematic Apperception Test involves the presentation of
      ten stories
D.   traits show considerable personal consistency over time
E.   the Rorschach inkblot test is a projective technique

25. Autosomal recessive causes of mental handicap include:

A.   tuberous sclerosis
B.   galactosaemia
C.   Lesch–Nyhan syndrome
D.   Apert syndrome
E.   Lawrence–Moon–Biedl syndrome

26. With regard to the neuropsychological maturation of infants:

A.   most infants smile by six weeks old
B.   there is an order of developmental changes that does not vary
      between children
C.   neonates can see an object held 30 centimetres in front of them
D.   early deprivation has lasting effects on motor skills
E.   sitting without support is accomplished by 80% of
      six-month-old infants

27. With regard to the serotonergic system in the CNS:

A.   the availability of tryptophan is rate limiting in the synthesis of
      serotonin
B.   there is evidence that increased CSF 5-HIAA may be a
      predictor of suicide and poor impulse control
C.   most of the 5-HT released in the CNS originates from the cells
      of the Raphe nuclei of the brainstem and mid-brain
D.   the system includes at least 8 receptor subtypes widely
      distributed throughout the CNS and the periphery
E.   depression may be precipitated by reserpine inhibiting
      tryptophan hydroxylase

28. The following drug effects on dopamine (DA) neurotransmission are correct:

A. amphetamines inhibit DA re-uptake from the synaptic cleft
B. tetrabenazine decreases synthesis of DA
C. reserpine causes irreversible depletion of DA from presynaptic vesicles
D. bromocriptine increases the release of DA from the presynaptic vesicles
E. tranylcypromine reduces the degradation and re-uptake of DA

29. The spinothalamic pathway:

A. terminates in the nucleus gracilis and nucleus cuneatus
B. relays sensations of pain and temperature
C. has its first-order neurones in the ventral root ganglion
D. crosses the midline at the point of entry of the root fibres
E. is particularly vulnerable to expanding central cord lesions

30. The following statements are true:

A. noradrenaline is formed by the hydroxylation of L-tryptophan
B. 20% of total body serotonin is in the CNS
C. side-effects produced by excess dopamine include diarrhoea and cramps
D. lysergic acid (LSD) is a 5-HT receptor agonist in the CNS
E. monoamine oxidase inhibitors are contraindicated when using tryptophan

31. Gamma amino butyric acid (GABA):

A. is absent from the peripheral nervous system
B. is found in high concentrations in the hippocampus
C. is released by the cerebellar Purkinje cells
D. may inhibit experimentally induced aggression
E. hyperpolarises its target cells and inhibits the influx of chloride ions

32. Excitatory neurotransmitters include:

A. glycine
B. serotonin
C. glutamic acid
D. acetyl choline
E. dopamine

33. The effects of benzodiazepines include:

A. an increase in fast beta activity on the EEG
B. increased serum levels of cortisol and prolactin
C. a reduction in the discharges of the limbic system causing anterograde amnesia
D. an increase in stage 4 sleep
E. closure of the chloride ion channels on the post-synaptic receptors

34. In the ageing non-demented brain:

A. it is rare to find neurofibrillary tangles in the neocortex
B. glial cells decrease in size and number
C. the degree of cerebral atrophy correlates with the degree of intellectual decline
D. eosinophilic inclusions (Hirano bodies) occur mainly in the hippocampus
E. lipofuscin accumulates in relation to cell loss only

35. Neuropathological changes found in the brains of schizophrenic patients include:

A. a significant decrease in brain weight when compared with well-matched controls
B. enlargement of the left temporal horn of the lateral ventricle
C. ventricular enlargement only in patients with a history of perinatal trauma
D. a clear correlation between severity of defect state and structural abnormality
E. lack of correlation between length of illness and increased ventricular size

36. Features of right parietal lobe damage include:

A.   contralateral visuospatial neglect
B.   'spontaneous' pain
C.   visual agnosia
D.   contralateral deficit of joint position sense
E.   agraphaesthesia

37. In clozapine therapy:

A.   white cell count monitoring needs to be carried out weekly for as long as the therapy continues
B.   drowsiness is usually only experienced in the first few days of treatment
C.   extrapyramidal side-effects are less common than with phenothiazines
D.   epilepsy is an absolute contraindication
E.   prescriptions are only for inpatients

38. Rating scales:

A.   to measure locus of control were introduced by Rotter (1966)
B.   exist to measure the cognitive aspects of pain
C.   can be used to assess psychotherapy outcome, but not psychotherapy process
D.   such as the Life Event Scale (Paykel et al., 1971) rely on observer ratings of taped interviews about events
E.   such as the Bulimic Investigatory Test (Henderson and Freeman, 1987) are designed to measure bulimic behaviour in in-patients

39. In terms of validity:

    A.   construct validity is evaluated by investigating what qualities a test measures

    B.   convergent validity is held to be established when measures that are predicted to be associated are found not to be related

    C.   divergent validity is where measures discriminate between other measures of related constructs

    D.   face validity can be determined by statistical methods

    E.   cross-validation may involve assessing criterion validity in different populations

40. In research psychophysiology:

    A.   the P300 is an early event-related potential

    B.   the P300 occurs 300 nanoseconds after the stimulus which generates it

    C.   the P300 may show different patterns of change in Alzheimer's dementia and the Korsakoff state

    D.   galvanic skin responses are measured in non-thermoregulatory areas of skin

    E.   penile plethysmography has demonstrated a relative reduction of nocturnal penile tumescence in depressed men

41. In the neurobiology of the ageing brain:

    A.   neurofibrillary tangles occur only in Alzheimer's disease

    B.   neurofibrillary tangles are paired helical filaments

    C.   neurofibrillary tangles are composed mainly of tau proteins

    D.   amyloid is deposited in senile plaques and in cerebral vasculature in Alzheimer's disease

    E.   the amyloid precursor protein gene has been located on chromosome 18

42. In severe depressive illness:

A. cortisol hypersecretion often occurs
B. the dexamethasone suppression test is highly specific
C. 5-HT$_1$ receptors are found to be significantly increased at post-mortem
D. platelet 5-HT uptake is significantly reduced
E. basal fasting serum growth hormone concentrations are greatly decreased

43. Alpha (α) adrenoreceptor agonists include:

A. α-methyldopa
B. noradrenaline
C. chlorpromazine
D. clonidine
E. isoproterenol

44. Cortical neuropeptides include:

A. angiotensin
B. cholecystokinin
C. neurotensin
D. enkephalin
E. vasoactive intestinal peptide

45. In the normal EEG:

A. alpha rhythm is maximal over the occiput
B. delta waves become more obvious with relaxation and drowsiness
C. beta activity attenuates when an individual engages in mental activity and reappears when the eyes are opened
D. spike waves commonly appear during sleep in children
E. theta activity does not appear

46. Amnesia for a criminal offence:

A. most commonly occurs in homicide cases
B. can occur if the individual is floridly psychotic
C. in multiple personality is usually fabricated
D. is invariable if the crime is committed during an automatism
E. negates the intent for the offence if associated with alcohol intoxication

47. A child of four shows the following characteristics according to Piaget:

A. capability to think symbolically
B. mastery of concept of conservation of numbers but not mass
C. egocentricity in approach to events
D. reasoning based on inner mechanisms not on observation of the real world
E. ability to initiate activities and see them through

48. Cocaine:

A. once absorbed is rapidly broken down by esterases
B. depresses synthesis of dopamine when repeatedly used
C. promotes learning of secondary associations between cocaine taking and cues for use
D. is well-absorbed through the oral mucosa
E. may be used in the palliative treatment of terminal cancer

49. The hypothalamus:

A. has osmoreceptors to detect increased osmotic pressure in the carotid blood supply
B. has output fibres in the principal mamillar fasciculus
C. includes the mamillary nucleus
D. controls the neurosecretory cells of the adenohypophysis via the neurohypophysial tract
E. receives inputs from the hippocampus

50. Clozapine:

A. occupies D_1 receptors to a greater extent than other neuroleptics
B. inhibits apomorphine
C. interacts with warfarin
D. is serotonergic
E. does not cause akathisia

MCQ Paper Two

Answers

1. A = T, B = T, C = T, D = F, E = F.

In the Continuous Performance Test a computer screen is used. The subject has to respond to predesignated stimuli on the screen that are presented transiently amongst rapidly changing random stimuli. Cognitive performance on a variety of tests, including short-term recall memory, is impaired in schizophrenia (Rund, 1989). Abnormalities in smooth pursuit eye movement (SPEM) occur independent of medication in schizophrenia and bipolar affective disorder. SPEMs are abnormal in up to 50% of first-degree relatives of patients with schizophrenia raising the question that SPEM may be a trait marker. The Wisconsin Card Sorting Test is more a measure of task planning, execution and perseveration in frontal lobe disorders. The WCST is also abnormal in chronic schizophrenia where there are also defects in conceptual shifts (as seen particularly in paranoid schizophrenia).

Rund BR (1989) Distractibility and recall capability in schizophrenics: a four year longitudinal study of stability in cognitive performance. Schizophrenia Res, 2, 265-75.
Rund BR, Landrø NI (1990) Information processing: a new model for understanding cognitive disturbances in psychiatric patients. Acta Psychiatr Scand, 81, 305-16.

2. A = F, B = F, C = T, D = T, E = T.

George Kelly's personal construct theory supposes that man is a scientist who hypothesises about the world and tests out those hypotheses. Based on these experiments, man develops personal constructs which are bipoles, e.g. good self – bad self, trust vs. not-trust. Certain of these constructs are more important than others and are termed core constructs. These are so important that an individual may kill him or herself rather than compromise these core constructs. The creativity cycle refers to the procedure whereby artists or scientists create new things. The initial phase might involve loosening constructs to generate new hypotheses or forms of music or stories, but any new combination of constructs so formed may have to be tightened so that the ideas are given an understandable form. For instance in order to generate a new story, a novelist might have to create a new character and cast about for a suitable theme. Once these have been generated, though, the constructs involved need to be tightened and the whole given a more consistent form, e.g a novel which contains the plot and character but which has a defined form, i.e. beginning, middle and end.

Kelly GA (1955) The Psychology of Personal Constructs: Vols 1 and 2. New York, Norton.

3.

A = T, B = F, C = F, D = F, E = F.

The Bedford College method of assessing life events takes into account the social context of that event in measuring the impact on the individual, unlike many life-event scales and schedules. The event is assessed in terms of its *meaning* for the individual rather than how the individual reports that they felt at the time. The judgements and severity ratings are made by a trained team based on the context of a lengthy and detailed interview.

Brown GW, Harris T (1978) Social Origins of Depression. London, Tavistock.

4.

A = F, B = F, C = T, D = T, E = F.

80% of night-time sleep is filled by orthodox or non-REM sleep. Awakenings from paradoxical sleep (REM) may yield descriptions of vivid dreams. Sleep deprivation in excess of 60 hours may stimulate illusions, hallucinations and persecutory ideas. During slow-wave sleep, growth hormone release is increased. Almost all cases of narcolepsy have the HLA type DR2 (cf 25% of the general population).

Oswald I (1980) Sleep. Harmondsworth, Penguin.
Waterhouse J (1993) Circadian rhythms. Br Med J, 306, 448-51.

5.

A = T, B = F, C = T, D = F, E = T.

Prosopagnosia implies an impairment in facial recognition. Constructional apraxias can occur in left and right hemispheric lesions, but there is a *qualitative* difference between right and left hemispheric constructional apraxias. Right hemisphere lesions lead to a so-called 'exploded' diagram, whereas left hemisphere lesions produce 'oversimplified' diagrams.

McCarthy RA, Warrington EK (1990) Cognitive Neuropsychology. California, Academic Press.

6. A = T, B = T, C = T, D = F, E = T.

Reliability across time, between diagnosticians and between reporting sources (e.g. patient and informant) is important. Specificity implies that diagnostic elements should be discrete and to some extent mutually exclusive. Internal consistency implies that the core symptoms should 'hang together' as measured by the covariance of the elements. A diagnosis becomes a 'meaningless label' if it has no external validity i.e. a diagnostic category must have some value in terms of epidemiological characteristics, aetiology, prognosis and treatment.

Werry JS (1992) Child psychiatric disorders: are they classifiable? Br J Psychiatr, 161, 472-80.

7. A = F, B = T, C = F, D = F, E = T.

The central tendency is the point in a distribution around which other scores tend to cluster. The probability that a given result could be caused by sampling error is called the statistical significance. The Z-score is a score minus the mean divided by the standard deviation. An ordinal measure has categories that are ranked, but not in terms of equal size. A nominal measure has distinct categories that cannot be ranked.

8. A = F, B = F, C = T, D = F, E = F.

The Parental Bonding Instrument is a 25-item questionnaire given to patients who rate statements about their mother and father. Neurotic depressives give lower care scores and higher control scores to their parents.

Parker G, Tupling H, Brown LB (1979) A parental bonding instrument. Br J Med Psychol, 52, 1-10.

9. A = F, B = T, C = F, D = T, E = T.

Simple classical conditioning can occur in cases of organic amnesia. Amnesia can be caused by independent lesions of the medial temporal lobes; midline diencephalon; and cholinergic basal forebrain (Mayes, 1991). Hippocampal lesions produce a mild retrograde amnesia affecting only a few years back. Anterograde and retrograde memory may be affected in the Wernicke-Korsakoff syndrome (Parkin, 1991).

Mayes A (1991) Amnesia: lesion location and functional deficit. Psychol Med, 21, 293-7.

Parkin AJ (1991) The relationship between anterograde and retrograde amnesia in alcoholic Wernicke–Korsakoff syndrome. Psychol Med, 21, 11-14.

10. A=F, B=F, C=T, D=T, E=F.

Prader–Willi syndrome is a rare cause (1%) of cases of mental handicap. Prader–Willi cases are characterised by hypotonia, hyperphagia, and hypogenitalism (Butler, 1990). Huntington's disease has been repeatedly found to have an earlier age of onset if inherited from the male (Bird et al., 1974), and has been cited as an example of genomic imprinting. In genomic imprinting the severity of expression of a genetic disease is affected by whether the particular chromosomes are derived from maternal or paternal sources. The effect is also cited in neurofibromatosis, myotonic dystrophy and cerebellar ataxia (Hall, 1990).

Bird ED, Caro AJ, Pilling JB (1974) A sex-related factor in the inheritance of Huntington's chorea. Ann Hum Genet, 37, 255-60.
Butler MG (1990) Prader–Willi syndrome: current understanding of cause and diagnosis. Am J Med Genet. 35, 319-32.
Hall JG (1990) Genomic imprinting: review and relevance to human disease. Am J Hum Genet, 35, 314-18.

11. A=F, B=T, C=T, D=T, E=F.

A type 1 error occurs when the p value is so small that the null hypothesis can be rejected, but the association being studied arises by chance. A type 2 error occurs when a real association is missed because the variation is too large for the sample size. Confidence intervals are used in an attempt to minimise these problems in interpreting results. The association between some factor and a disease may be because the factor causes the disease, or it may be because the disease causes the factor, or some other intermediary link. A confounder is some factor associated with both the disease and the 'exposure' that can lead to a spurious association. For instance, if depression is found to be associated with smoking; is the smoking having direct effects on the brain, or might it be some confounding variable, e.g. chronic bronchitis? Multivariate analyses are suitable for a variety of study designs.

Lewis G, Mann A (1992) Epidemiology. In: Weller M, Eysenck M (eds), The Scientific Basis of Psychiatry. London, Saunders.

12. A=F, B=T, C=F, D=F, E=F.

The absolute threshold is the lowest intensity of a stimulus that can be detected. In dichotic listening, two different messages are presented simultaneously through headphones and the subject is asked to pay attention to only one of the messages. The 'unattended' message is still processed by the brain though and attention can switch if its contents are of more interest, e.g. if the subject's name is mentioned in the 'unattended' message (Treisman, 1969). The Stroop effect is where the names of colours are printed in hues different from the names. The subject is then asked to go through the colours of the *inks* saying which colours they are. We are accustomed to reading out the words as soon as they are seen, and so this automatic processing interferes with the more conscious task. Cortical area, adjacent to the primary visual cortex carry out separate, parallel image processing. These separate analyses are integrated with other analyses in the inferotemporal brain area. In reading, 'bottom-up' processing involves a step-by-step analysis, each step having to be completed before the next. In 'top-down' processing there is feedback from the later stages of interpretation; so that expectations of what a word might represent affect how it is perceived.

Treisman AM (1969) Strategies and models of selective attention. Psychol Rev, 76, 282-99.

13. A=F, B=F, C=T, D=F, E=T.

In the notation for gene location, the first item is the chromosome number, the second whether the gene is on the short or long arm and thirdly the segment number of the arm where the gene is. In terms of which arm the gene is on, 'p' denotes the short arm and 'q' denotes the long arm. Recombinant DNA can be produced by inserting 'foreign' DNA into plasmid or cosmid DNA and then getting these to replicate in bacteria. In genetic linkage studies, the log of the odds score (lod score) for various values of the recombination fraction, indicates significant linkage if it is greater than 3. In analysing pedigrees of manic depression the lod score has been found to be very sensitive to diagnostic errors such that data may be misinterpreted and the wrong conclusions made (Kelsoe et al., 1989).

Kelsoe JR, Ginns EI, Egeland JA, et al. (1989) Re-evaluation of linkage relationship between chromosome 11p loci and the gene for bipolar affective disorder in the Old Order Amish. Nature, 342, 238-43.

14. A = F, B = T, C = T, D = F, E = F.

Validity is an assessment of whether a test or scale measures what it is supposed to. If there is a high correlation between the test score and the quality it is supposed to measure, then the test is said to be valid. Reliability is concerned with whether the scale or test can achieve consistent results. Concurrent validity compares test scores with established criteria or tests performed at the same time. The Brief Psychiatric Rating Scale is an intensity scale, widely used to assess change during treatment trials. The Hamilton Rating Scale has had high inter-rater reliability scores of about 0.9 (Hamilton, 1976). Average rating scales achieve inter-rater reliability scores of approximately 0.6.

Hamilton M (1976) Comparative value of rating scales. Br J Clin Pharmacol, Suppl., 58-60.

15. A = T, B = F, C = T, D = F, E = F.

In 1955 and subsequently, Asch published results of an experiment into groups and an individual's decision making. To test this Asch set up a card with a single vertical line on it. Some distance away he set up a second card with three lines of different length upon it. Volunteer groups were asked to say which of the three was the same as the original. However, of the groups, only one individual was the subject. Unbeknownst to him or her, the rest of the group were not bona fide volunteers but had been previously primed to disagree with the true subject. The analysis looked at whether the individual's decision was swayed by the group. Asch found that 75% of individuals tend to conform with the group decision on line length, even if they suspect the group is wrong. A minority stick out for what they believe. The group's effect in producing such conformity peaked when the individual was confronted by three opposing views. Adding further opposition did not produce a cumulative effect. If the individual was joined by another partner with the same dissenting voice, then yielding to the group diminished.

Asch SE (1955) Opinions and social pressure. Sci Am, 193, 31-5.

16. A = T, B = F, C = F, D = T, E = F.

Lloyd Homme introduced the concept of coverant behaviour, a contraction of covert and operant, to describe the mental events or behaviours that mimic observable operant behaviour, such as intrusive thoughts. BF Skinner wrote an account of the acquisition of language and the development of thought in *Verbal Behaviour* (1957). Skinner has made numerous contributions to behavioural psychology, including operant conditioning, the Skinner box, and shaping where behaviour is shaped by controlling the responses the environment makes to particular behaviours. John B Watson almost started the behavioural school of psychology by focusing on observable behaviours. Prior to his intervention, psychologists had been focused mainly on mental processes and ideas regarding consciousness.

Partial re-inforcement occurs where a response is re-inforced only some of the time. This makes it less likely to be extinguished when re-inforcement eventually stops than if continuous re-inforcement had been previously used (Humphrey, 1939)

Homme LE (1965) Perpectives in psychology: xxiv. Control of coverants: the operants of the mind. Psychol Rec, 15, 501.
Humphrey LG (1939) The effect of random alternation of re-inforcement on the acquisition and extinction of conditioned eyelid reactions. J Exp Psychol, 25, 141-58.

17. A = F, B = F, C = T, D = T, E = F.

Support for a universal National Health Service is highest amongst social classes I and II. Only 30% of the people feel that medical treatment in hospitals could be higher quality. 54% of people are satisfied with outpatient services, but 79% are satisfied with ther General Practitioners. In 1987, 61% of 25–34-year-olds felt that homosexual relationships are always or mostly wrong. This attitude had become more prevalent over the years 1983–1987, with a 10% increase for male respondents and a 15% for women respondents. Right and wrong are seen as matters of degree. For instance, 36% of people would say that 'fiddling' travel expenses of £200 is 'seriously wrong' whereas only 15% would think that 'fiddling' £50 is 'seriously wrong'.

Jowell R, Witherspoon S, Brook L (eds) (1988) British Social Attitudes. 5th Report. Hants, Gower.

18. A = T, B = T, C = F, D = T, E = F.

Piaget called his program to study the development of children's intelligence 'genetic epistemology'. He described four stages of development of children's thought: sensori-motor, preoperational, concrete operations, and formal operational thought. Object constancy describes the ability to recognise the continued existence of an object even when it is out of the immediate arena of awareness. Preoperational children fail to appreciate the conservation of quantity when, say, a constant volume of liquid is poured from a tube of small diameter to a tube of wider diameter. It was Spearman (1863–1945), an English psychologist, who coined the two-factor theory of intelligence, involving a general intelligence (g), and a task-specific intelligence (s).

19. A = F, B = T, C = T, D = F, E = T.

The Registrar-General's classification has 6 occupational unit groups:
- I Professional
- II Intermediate
- III Skilled Occupations (Non-manual)
- III Skilled Occupations (Manual)
- IV Semi-skilled Occupations
- V Unskilled Occupations.

Goldthorpe's schema has 11 categories, including salariat, bourgeoisie, manual foreman, and working class.

Senile dementia of the Alzheimer type has been found to be more prevalent in the lowest classes (Sulkava et al., 1985), and within age groups higher rates have been found in persons with less education (Gurland et al., 1983) .

Gurland B, Copeland J, Kuriansky J, et al. (1983) The Mind and Mood of Aging. London, Croom Helm.
Sulkava R, et al. (1985) Prevalence of senile dementia in Finland. Neurology, 35, 1025-9.

20. A = F, B = F, C = T, D = F, E = T.

Post-mortem brain studies have suggested that there are increased concentrations of D2 receptors in schizophrenia; other studies have pointed to neuroleptic administration as a cause of this finding.

Iversen LL (1985) Mechanism of action of antipsychotic drugs: retrospect and prospect. In: Iversen SD (ed), Psychpharmacology: Recent Advances and Future Prospects. Oxford, Oxford Medical Publications.

Owen F, et al. (1985) Dopamine (D2) receptors and schizophrenia. In: Iversen SD (ed), Psychpharmacology: Recent Advances and Future Prospects. Oxford, Oxford Medical Publications.

21. All false.

The incidence rate is the number of episodes of ill health begun, or people becoming ill in a specified time over the number exposed to risk at the midpoint of the period. The average duration of the illness can be calculated using the point prevalence rate divided by the incidence rate. The point prevalence rate refers to a specific point in time not over a period of time. A specific rate looks at particular sections of the population in terms of age or occupation, unlike a crude rate which looks at an essentially undifferentiated population.

22. A = F, B = F, C = F, D = F, E = T.

Parametric methods depend on assumptions made about distributions, e.g. Student's t distribution. Non-parametric methods are distribution-free, e.g the chi-squared distribution which is used for categorical data.

Altman DG (1991) Practical Statistics for Medical Research. London, Chapman and Hall.

23. A = T, B = F, C = F, D = F, E = T.

Studies using metanalyis have found head injury to be associated with later idiopathic dementia (Anthony and Aboraya, 1992). Heavy alcohol consumption has been linked to later dementia, but as yet this is not a consistent finding (Gallo and Anthony, 1992). As far as family history of affective disorder is concerned, 13% of those with major depressive disorder aged over 60 had first-degree relatives with affective disorder compared with 29% of depressives aged less than 60 (Brodaty et al., 1991). In 1987, Torrey reviewed 70 epidemiological studies and found a 50-fold difference in rates, although the majority of rates fell into a range of between 2 and 5 per 1000. Such differences might be explained by differences in diagnostic criteria and other methodologies making direct comparison of studies difficult, but Torrey felt that overall the magnitude of differences in 'reliable' prevalence rates was ten-fold. Opjordsmoen (1991) has reported a very long-term outcome study of schizophrenia in Norway and found that men had more negative symptoms and women had more affective and paranoid symptoms, which echoed Goldtsein et al.'s proposed subtypes of schizophrenia (1990) in which one was characterised by winter birth, flat affect, poor premorbid history, and a second with dysphoria and paranoid delusions.

Anthony JC, Aboraya A (1992) The epidemiology of selected mental disorders in later life. In: Handbook of Mental Health and Aging, 2nd Edn. New York, Academic Press.
Brodaty H, Peters K, Boyce P, et al. (1991) Age and depression. J Affect Disorder, 23, 137-49.
Gallo JJ, Anthony JC (1992) Epidemiologic studies: risk factors and clinical features. Curr Opin Psychiatr, 5, 548-53.
Goldstein JM, Santangelo SL, Simpson JC, Tsuang MT. The role of gender in identifying subtypes of schizophrenia. Schizophrenia Bull, 16, 263-75.
Opjordmoen S (1991) Long-term clinical outcome of schizophrenia with special reference to gender differences. Acta Psychiatr Scand, 83, 307-13.
Torrey EF (1987) Prevalence studies in schizophrenia. Br J Psychiatr, 150, 598-608.

24. A = T, B = F, C = F, D = T, E = T.

The Minnesota Multiphasic Personality Inventory (MMPI) appeared in 1940 and is an example of a self-administered inventory of 550 items. These items can be organised into various scales, which include scales for conversion hysteria, depression, paranoia, schizophrenia, masculinity/femininity, introversion, neurosis, hypochondria, and psychopathic deviate. These scales are organised to give a graphical score profile. Lying scales are also incorporated into the MMPI. The MMPI was developed on a psychiatric population. The California Personality Inventory was developed on and for a 'normal' population. The Thematic Apperception Test (TAT) and the Rorschach Inkblot Test are examples of projective techniques. The TAT involves the presentation of pictures of various scenes which the subject must describe in terms of what is happening, what happened before and what the outcome will be. Personality traits generally show considerable consistency over time (Block, 1971).

Block J (1971) Lives Through Time. California, Bancroft.

25. A = F, B = T, C = F, D = F, E = T.

Tuberous sclerosis is an autosomal dominant condition. Galactosaemia involves a deficiency of galactose 1-phosphate uridyl transferase, resulting in retardation, hepatomegaly and cataracts. An galactose-free diet is effective if started early. Lesch–Nyhan syndrome is an example of an X-linked recessive disorder. Lesch–Nyhan syndrome is a disorder of purine metabolism resulting in excess uric acid production. It is characterised by self-mutilation, mental retardation and involuntary movements. Apert syndrome is an autosomal dominant condition with skull malformation, syndactyly and variable degrees of retardation. Lawrence–Moon–Biedl syndrome involves moderate retardation, pigmentary retinopathy, hypogenitalism and polydactyly.

BG

26. A = T, B = T, C = T, D = F, E = F.

The maturational processes of children are mainly determined by heredity. Environmental factors may accelerate or retard development but the order of the developmental stages does not vary. Infants learn to focus at one month, but neonates can see objects at 30 centimetres from birth. Early deprivation has been shown to have permament effects on emotional and intellectual skills, but not on motor skills. Sitting without support is accomplished by 50% of children at six months.

27. A = T, B = F, C = T, D = T, E = F.

Knowledge of the serotonergic system is increasing rapidly and currently 8 receptor subtypes are identified. Numerous studies have shown that significant decreases in brain 5-HT concentrations and reduced CSF 5-HIAA in depressed patients may be predictors of aggression and suicidality. Reserpine affects 5-HT stores in the nerve terminal and reduces the availability of 5-HT. Theoretically dietary deficiency of tryptophan may impact on brain serotonergic synthesis.

(1992) J Clin Psychiatr. 53, 10 (suppl.).

28. A = F, B = F, C = T, D = F, E = T.

Amphetamines have a variety of effects on DA transmission, including increased release of DA from pre-synaptic vesicles, inhibition of re-uptake and inhibition of DA degradation by monoamine oxidase.

Tetrabenazine reversibly depletes DA storage whereas reserpine has an irreversible effect on this process. Bromocriptine is a dopamine agonist acting mainly at post-synaptic D2 receptors. Tranylcypromine and related drugs decrease the degradation of DA by inhibiting MAO. Tranylcypromine also reduces the uptake of DA.

29. A = F, B = T, C = F, D = F, E = T.

The spinothalamic tract terminates in the ventro post lateral nucleus of the thalamus. The first-order neurones have cell bodies in the dorsal root ganglia. The tract crosses one or two segments above the level of entry of the root fibres. As the tract crosses the anterior white commissure, it is vulnerable to central expanding lesions, e.g. syringomyelia

Barr ML, Kiernan JA (1988) The Human Nervous System, 5th Edn. Philadelphia, Lippincott.

30. A = F, B = F, C = T, D = T, E = F.

Serotonin is formed by the hydroxylation of L-tryptophan to 5-hydroxytryptophan which is then decarboxylated to 5-hydroxytryptamine. Less than two per cent of total body serotonin is in the CNS. Diarrhoea and cramps can be caused by DA and 5-HT. LSD can have 5-HT antagonistic effects peripherally. The dose of l-tryptophan needs to be reduced when used with irreversible MAOIs and should be discontinued if blurred vision or headache occur.

31. A = T, B = T, C = T, D = T, E = F.

GABA is a major inhibitory neurotransmitter and produces its effect by hyperpolarisation of the target cell. Some types of spontaneous and experimentally induced aggression can be inhibited by potentiation of GABA inhibitory control. GABA is found in high concentrations in the hiipocampus. GABA is released by the Golgi and basket cells and the cerebellar Purkinje cells.

32. A = F, B = F, C = T, D = T, E = F.

Inhibitory neurotransmitters include noradrenaline, serotonin, dopamine, GABA and endorphins. Excitatory transmitters include acetylcholine and glutamic acid.

Mackay AVP, Iversen LL (1992) Neurotransmitters and schizophrenia. In: Weller M, Eysenck M (eds), The Scientific Basis of Psychiatry. London, Saunders.

33. A = T, B = T, C = T, D = F, E = F.

Benzodiazepines increase the seizure threshold. This action involves GABA as does its effect on increasing chloride ion influx. Benzodiazepines decrease stage 4 and REM sleep and, following withdrawal, rebound REM with disturbed sleep may occur. Benzodiazepines decrease the discharge of spinal and limbic neurones.

34. A = T, B = F, C = F, D = T, E = F.

Features of the neuropathology of SDAT can be found in the normal ageing non-demented brain. Cerebral atrophy is very common after the age of 60 when ventricular enlargement tends to occur. The correlation with intellectual decline is poor. Hirano bodies and features of Pick's disease may occur. Lipofuscin can accumulate in the absence of cell loss. In SDAT, plaques are distributed throughout the cortical layers whereas in the normal ageing brain they tend to be restricted to the superficial layers.

35. A = T, B = T, C = F, D = F, E = T.

A number of studies have shown a significant decrease in brain weight, length and volume in schizophrenic patients compared with controls. Ventricular enlargement has been demonstrated in post-mortem studies particularly of the left temporal lobe. Ventricular enlargement is evident in patients with positive and negative symptoms. The clinical correlates of structural change are unclear but the extent of the structural changes appear to correlate with the degree of cognitive impairment. Unlike neurodegenerative conditions there is a lack of correlation between the length of the illness and the increased ventricular size.

Roberts GW (1991) Schizophrenia, a neuropathological perspective. Br J Psychiatr, 158, 8-17.

36. A = T, B = F, C = F, D = T, E = T.

Features of right (non-dominant) parietal lobe damage include contralateral neglect in which the patient may ignore deficits on his left hand side. His or her writing may be indecipherable as it is crowded on the right side of the page and, when reading, he or she will ignore what is on the left hand side of the page. Spontaneous pain is a feature of the thalamic syndrome. Visual agnosia, the failure to recognise objects by sight although retaining the capacity perhaps to recognise them in another sensory modality, is regarded as a feature of bilateral damage to the posterior cerebral hemispheres. Contralateral defects of joint position sense, tactile localisation, and two-point discrimination can occur. Agraphaesthesia is the inability to recognise numbers or letters written, say, on the palm of the hand.

37. A=F, B=T, C=T, D=F, E=F.

Clozapine therapy demands that white cell counts are monitored weekly for the first 18 weeks and fortnightly thereafter. As clozapine has less affinity for D1 receptors than phenothiazines it causes fewer extrapyramidal side-effects. Patients with epilepsy on clozapine require very close monitoring and a gradual build-up of the dose. Clozapine can only be dispensed by hospital pharmacies at present and all patients have to be registered with manufacturers for their patient monitoring service. Although patients need to begin therapy in hospital, ongoing community treatment is possible with adequate monitoring arrangements.

AO'H

38. A=T, B=T, C=F, D=F, E=F.

Rotter (1966) introduced the concept of the internal locus of control where events, feelings and experiences are perceived as attributable to personal action. Where they are perceived as beyond personal responsibility this is an external locus of control. The McGill pain questionnaire records the severity of pain and its cognitive and affective aspects. In psychotherapy research, scales have been developed to look at process, e.g. where the therapist and patient rate the session as a whole, or where experts rate audio or video tapes of sessions. The Life Event Scale (Paykel et al., 1971) is a 61-item scale in which life changes and events are scored according to their presumed stress values. The Bulimic Investigatory Test is designed to identify binge-eaters in epidemiological surveys.

Henderson M, Freeman CPL (1987) A self-rating scale for bulimia, the 'BITE'. Br J Psychiatr, 100, 18-24.
Paykel ES, Prusoff BA, Uhlenhuth EH (1971) Scaling of life events. Arch Gen Psychiatr, 25, 340-7.
Rotter JB (1966) Generalised expectancies for internal versus external control of re-inforcement. Psychol Monogr, 80, 609.

39. A = T, B = F, C = F, D = F, E = T.

The American Psychological Association (1954) stated that "construct validity is evaluated by investigating what qualities a test measures". Convergent validity occurs when measures that are predicted to be associated are found to be related (i.e. measure the same thing), as opposed to divergent validity where measures successfully discriminate between unrelated constructs. Face validity is a judgement of whether some test measures what it is supposed to measure.

American Psycholgical Association (1954) Technical recommendations for psychological tests and diagnostic techniques. Psychol Bull, Suppl 51, part 2, 1-38.

40. A = F, B = F, C = T, D = T, E = T.

The P300 is a late event-related potential. Early event-related potentials occur within 20 ms of stimulation. Later event-related potentials occur after 70 ms. The P300 occurs 300 milliseconds after auditory, visual and somatosensory stimuli. The latency of the P300 increases with the difficulty of the task required of the subject and the amplitude increases with the unexpectedness of the stimuli.

Alzheimer's patients have been reported to have delayed latency and reduced P300 amplitude, but the Korsakoff group has been reported not to differ significantly from controls in terms, despite severe memory impairment. Thase et al. (1987) noted a reduction in nocturnal penile tumescence in depressed men.

Blackwood DHR, Muir WJ (1990) Cognitive brain potentials and their application. Br J Psychiatr, 157 (suppl 9), 96-101.
Thase ME, et al. (1987) Nocturnal penile tumescence in depressed men. Am J Psychiatr, 143, 478-82.

41. A = F, B = T, C = T, D = T, E = F.

Neurofibrillary tangles are more frequent in Alzheimer's disease, but do occur in other conditions and in the normal aged brain. The amyloid precursor protein gene has been located on chromosome 21.

Levy AI, Sisodia SS, Price DL (1992) Advances in the molecular neurobiology of Alzheimer's disease. Curr Opin Psychiatr, 5, 98-102.

42. A = T, B = F, C = F, D = F, E = F.

The dexamethasone suppression test is abnormal in some cases of severe depression, but is also abnormal in a variety of other conditions. With regard to research on 5-HT$_1$ receptors, what evidence there is suggests that there is no significant difference in the number of recptors in 'depressed' brains at post-mortem using standard ligand binding techniques (McKeith et al., 1987). There is some evidence to suggest that there are increases in 5-HT$_2$ receptor density in depression, but the body of evidence is not unequivocal. There is clearly much work to be done before a satisfactory conclusion is reached, especially as there are at least seven 5-HT receptor subtypes to work on. The use of platelets as models for neurons has focused on neurotransmitter uptake. Work on platelet 5-HT uptake in various brain areas has failed to show any convincing difference in depression to date (Bech et al., 1988).

Bech P, Aplov L, Gastpar M (1988) WHO pilot study on the validity of imipramine platelet receptor binding sites as a biological marker of endogenous depression. Pharmacopsychiatry, 21, 147-50.
Power AC, Cowen PJ (1992) Fluoxetine and suicidal behaviour. Br J Psychiatr. 61, 735-41.

43. A = F, B = T, C = F, D = T, E = F.

44. A = F, B = T, C = F, D = F, E = T.
Within the brain, neuropeptides exist at a much lower concentrations than classical neurotransmitters. The highest concentrations of neuropeptides occur in the hypothalamopituitary system.

BG

45. A = T, B = T, C = F, D = F, E = F.
Alpha rhythm is prominent over the occiput – it is accentuated by eye closure and attenuated by opening the eyes. Delta waves are diffusely distributed and normally seen only in sleeping adults and in children. Beta activity is principally frontocentral and increases with relaxation. Spike waves are invariably abnormal. Theta activity may appear transiently in about 15% of the population. Lambda single sharp waves are usually associated with visual scanning.

46. A = T, B = T, C = F, D = F, E = F.
Most studies have found that amnesia is a common finding in those charged with homicide and violent crimes. Amnesia in multiple personality is usually regarded as being due to a hysterical dissociation. Each persona has an amnesia for the other personae. Amnesia will only negate the intent if the intoxication was so severe that the accused could not form the necessary intent for the offence in question.

47. A = T, B = F, C = T, D = T, E = F.

A four-year-old child will be in Piaget's pre-operational stage of cognitive development, the characteristics of which include egocentrism, animism, and precausal logic. The child can think symbolically. Precausal logic is not scientific logic and is based on the child's inner representation of the world. The concept of conservation is associated with the concrete operational phase. Conservation of numbers may be attaned by the age of six. The ability to initiate activities is part of Erikson's 3rd stage of man (initiative versus guilt).

AO'H

48. A = T, B = T, C = T, D = F, E = T.

Cocaine taking rapidly links reward with secondary cues. These associated cues are very difficult to unlearn, so that environmental factors such as objects (like needles), people, occasions or places may trigger the association and cue cocaine abuse. Cocaine is poorly absorbed through the oral mucosa, only one per cent of the dose being absorbed. Intranasal absorption is higher, but still only 5%. Cocaine forms part of the traditional Brompton cocktail, used in some terminal care cases (opiates, alcohol, and cocaine).

Strang J, Johns A, Caan W (1993) Cocaine in the UK – 1991. Br J Psychiatr, 162, 1-13.

49. A = T, B = T, C = T, D = F, E = T.

Osmoreceptors in the perinuclear areas stimulate cells of the supraoptic and periventricular nuclei to stop the release of antidiuretic hormone. The neurohypophysial tract has neural connections with the posterior pituitary rather than the adenohypophysis (anterior pituitary).

50. A = T, B = F, C = T, D = F, E = F.

Clozapine occupies a relatively low number of D_2 receptors compared with a high D_1 receptor occupancy. Clozapine is a potent α-adrenoceptor blocker and a serotonin blocker. Clozapine is protein-bound, like warfarin, hence the interaction.

McKenna PJ, Bailey PE (1993) The strange story of clozapine. Br J Psychiatr, 162, 32-7.

BG

MCQ Paper Three

Clinical Topics (MRCPsych Part II)
One-and-a-half hours
50 questions

1. The fragile-X syndrome:

A. is associated with repetitions of the base sequence CGG at the fragile site
B. accounts for up to 5% of all cases of mental retardation
C. may present with language delay
D. only affects males
E. is only diagnosed phenotypically

2. Males with schizophrenia (compared to females with schizophrenia):

A. have a similar age of onset
B. have fewer relapses
C. are more likely to have had abnormal premorbid intellectual and social functioning
D. are more likely to express negative symptoms such as social withdrawal
E. more often have structural brain abnormalities of neurodevelopmental origin

3. Deliberate self-harm:

A. as defined by Morgan (1979) does not include self-poisoning
B. is associated with bulimia nervosa
C. is a feature of DSM-III-R histrionic personality disorder
D. is associated with childhood sexual abuse
E. has been described as 'addictive'

4. **Epidemiological studies have yielded risk factors associated with the development of depression in adults which include:**

    A.   smoking
    B.   loneliness
    C.   loss of mother in early life
    D.   female sex
    E.   bereavement

5. **In the psychological management of depression:**

    A.   Beck postulated that treatment should focus on systematic cognitive errors
    B.   a combination of cognitive therapy with medication has not been shown to reduce the relapse rate
    C.   behaviour therapy aims to modify the performance of social behaviour
    D.   social skills training may prevent relapse
    E.   severe cases may benefit more than moderate cases

6. **Senile dementia of the Lewy body type:**

    A.   is much less common than multi-infarct dementia
    B.   is associated with inclusion bodies containing neurofilament and microtubule protein
    C.   usually involves loss of cells in the substantia nigra
    D.   often involves hallucinatory experience
    E.   only affects subcortical brain structures

7. **Epidemiological studies of eating disorders:**

    A.   have shown that the incidence of anorexia nervosa has increased in recent decades
    B.   sometimes use the EAT questionnaire
    C.   yield a consistent point prevalence of 20% for eating disorders in young British women
    D.   show that anorexic patients tend to avoid participating in surveys
    E.   suggest that different countries all have similar prevalence rates

8. In the history of psychiatry:

A. the York Retreat was founded by George Pinel
B. Morel proposed the degeneration theory
C. the Malleus Maleficarum was written by Galen
D. Eugen Bleuler argued that dementia praecox was a misnomer
E. the EEG was discovered in 1871

9. These names are correctly paired with their contributions to psychiatry:

A. Cerletti and ECT
B. Moniz and psychotherapy
C. Jellinek and pathological drinking
D. Russell and bulimia nervosa
E. Gage and frontal lobe syndrome

10. Damage to subcortical areas of the brain may result in:

A. Kleine–Levin syndrome
B. Kluver–Bucy syndrome
C. dysaesthesia
D. vegetative states
E. reduplicative paramnesia

11. Recognised features of Pick's disease include:

A. dyscalculia
B. predominantly parietal lobe damage
C. status spongiosus
D. reduced cerebrospinal fluid production
E. ventricular dilatation out of proportion to sulcal atrophy

12. Methods of reducing unwanted behaviour include:

A. response prevention
B. cue exposure
C. habit reversal
D. increasing delay between stimulus and response
E. stimulus control

13. Therapeutic factors in small group psychotherapy include:

A. instillation of hope
B. universality
C. vicarious learning
D. resistance
E. enmeshment

14. The following are characteristic features of systemic family therapy:

A. homeostasis
B. feedback loops
C. linear causality
D. subsystem boundaries
E. separation anxiety

15. To safely assess cerebral dominance:

A. sodium amytal can be injected into first one and then the other carotid arteries
B. verbal difficulties can be assessed after unilateral ECT
C. dichotic listening may be used
D. an EEG would show alpha-rhythm suppression during verbal thought
E. visual field studies cannot be used

16. Features of total institutions according to Goffman (1961) include:

A. encompassing tendencies
B. tightly scheduled activities
C. free communication between inmates and higher staff levels
D. people working, sleeping and playing in different environments
E. a split between a large managed group and a small supervisory group

17. Immigrants:

A.   face a culture shock, as defined by Toffler (1970)
B.   who are 'settlers' as defined by Rack (1986) tend to take a positive view of their new surroundings
C.   who are refugees have a lower psychiatric morbidity because they have a positive view of their new surroundings
D.   undergo a process of acculturation
E.   from the West Indies have been found to have a higher incidence of schizophrenia than British-born black people

18. According to Bentovim (1986) successful families should include:

A.   a model for socialisation
B.   models in the parents for sexual identity
C.   boundaries demarcating parents and children
D.   triangular relationship structures
E.   mutual dependency and investment

19. According to ICD-10, specific developmental disorders of scholastic skills include:

A.   specific speech articulation disorder
B.   specific reading disorder
C.   childhood autism
D.   specific disorder of arithmetical skills
E.   Rett's syndrome

20. Recognised features of hypothyroidism include:

A.   mennorrhagia
B.   muscle weakness
C.   generalised aches and pains
D.   delirium
E.   syncope

21. **The Wechsler Adult Intelligence Scale (WAIS):**

A.   includes a test of vocabulary
B.   involves a perceptual maze test
C.   has a sub-scale which assesses motor speed
D.   does not yield an intelligence quotient
E.   has a sub-test which asks the subject to say in what way two things are alike

22. **Which of the following statements regarding psychiatry and society are correct?**

A.   Voluntary patient status was first introduced in the UK in 1910
B.   Group therapy began with tuberculosis self-help groups in the 1950s
C.   Psychiatrists used to be termed 'alienists'
D.   North American States have had sterilisation programmes for the mentally ill and mentally handicapped
E.   'Life unworthy of Life' was a propaganda phrase used to describe psychiatric patients in Twentieth Century Europe

23. **Sexual problems:**

A.   such as impotence occur in 10% of 40 year olds
B.   are reported more often by men than women
C.   at the start of a marriage are associated with a higher risk of divorce
D.   and marital difficulties occur in about 10% of psychiatric clinic attenders
E.   in men are mainly due to erectile dysfunction

24. **In an initial interview with a 12-year-old girl who has possibly been sexually abused:**

A.   an anatomically correct doll should be used
B.   the detailed recall of past events is likely to be worse than in a fourteen year old
C.   the interviewer should educate the child as to the correct anatomical names for sexual organs
D.   enabling questions should not be used
E.   comforting gestures may be misinterpreted as threatening or provocative

25. In child psychotherapy, according to Winnicott:

A.   the mother–infant relationship is the paradigm for the analytic process

B.   an infant has a primary capacity for communication only after he or she begins to talk

C.   it is axiomatic that the work of the analysis is done by the patient

D.   the therapist should refrain from voicing interpretations

E.   the interpretation is only good for the patient if it is felt to have been created by him or her

26. Psychiatric manifestations of frontal lobe tumours:

A.   most commonly involve confusional states

B.   are commonly the first presenting feature of anteriorly placed frontal lobe tumours

C.   occur in greater frequency in gliomas than meningiomas

D.   commonly mimic affective disorder

E.   may be associated with incontinence

27. In the treatment of depression:

A.   bilateral ECT is more effective than unilateral

B.   monoamine oxidase (irreversible) inhibitors (MAOIs) are as effective overall as ECT in inpatients

C.   patients with reversed functional shift show a better response to traditional MAOIs

D.   controlled trials have demonstrated the superiority of tricyclic antidepressants over placebo in mild depression

E.   cognitive therapy is as effective as drug therapy in mild-to-moderate depression

28. Following a head injury, the following are true of memory disturbances that occur:

A.   the duration of retrograde amnesia predicts cognitive outcome

B.   the ability to learn new information is the slowest cognitive deficit to recover

C.   anterograde amnesia may persist for longer than post-traumatic amnesia

D.   following mild head injury, forgetfulness is a common complaint which clears after litigation

E.   loss of personal (episodic) memories is more suggestive of a psychogenic amnesia

29. In complex partial seizures:

A.   loss of consciousness does not occur

B.   spread to both hemispheres can occur with tonic–clonic seizures

C.   tumours are found in only 3% of adult patients

D.   speech automatisms are strongly related to a right temporal lobe focus

E.   forced thinking or thought blocking can occur as part of an aura

30. Writer's cramp:

A.   occurs more frequently in men than women

B.   is asymptomatic when the sufferer is not writing

C.   is characteristically associated with torsion dystonia

D.   tends to remit spontaneously

E.   may be associated with a prominent tremor

31. Phenylketonuria:

A.   has an incidence at birth of 1 in 10,000

B.   is transmitted in an autosomal dominant fashion

C.   is screened for using the Guthrie test on the first day of life

D.   is complicated by seizures in the majority of cases

E.   can only be treated by total exclusion of phenylalanine from the diet in childhood

32. In the episodic dyscontrol syndrome (intermittent explosive disorder):

    A.   individuals generally have a history of violence from early childhood

    B.   symptoms start to decline in the vast majority in the fourth decade

    C.   violent outbursts may be preceded by auras

    D.   EEG abnormalities are rarely described

    E.   chlordiazepoxide has been shown to be beneficial

33. In erectile impotence:

    A.   psychological therapy produces more significant improvements in sexual functioning than pharmacological therapy

    B.   intracavernosal injections of papaverine can lead to an improvement in spontaneous erectile function

    C.   suction devices are less effective than pharmacological therapy in producing an erection

    D.   the use of topical nitroglycerine may be limited by the development of headache in the patient's partner

    E.   priapism secondary to intrapenile injections can be succesfully treated by local injection of an α_2-adrenoceptor antagonist

34. The bereavement response in families with a handicapped child:

    A.   includes 'bargaining' and 'ego-centred work'

    B.   may lead to 'shopping around' in families fixated at the 'grief' stage

    C.   requires reality orientation to treat the 'fantasy' stage of acceptance

    D.   may lead to 'infantilisation' which is characterised by a failure to accept the child

    E.   precipitates transgenerational splits

35. Huntington's disease is characterised by:

A.   distractibility
B.   loss of alpha rhythms on EEG
C.   reduced levels of GABA and glutamic acid decarboxylase in the basal ganglia
D.   prominent language disorder in association with cognitive decline
E.   sparing of memory in comparison with other cognitive deficits as the dementia progresses

36. Characteristic features of opiate addication include:

A.   a marked alteration in the level of consciousness
B.   decreased appetite and reduced sexual urges
C.   a syndrome similar to delirium tremens within 36 hours of withdrawal
D.   flashbacks occurring months after the last use of the drug
E.   a paranoid psychosis with high doses

37. In treating depression:

A.   overall 40% of patients fail to respond to the initial antidepressant prescription
B.   more than 20% of patients are still depressed 2 years after the onset of the illness
C.   premorbid high neuroticism is associated with a poor prognosis
D.   which began more than six months prior to receiving treatment there is a poor prognosis
E.   which is refractory, lithium augmentation leads to a small increase in the response rate

38. Obsessive–compulsive disorder:

A.   is five times more common in women than men
B.   has a lifetime prevalence of 2–3% as reported in the Epidemiological Catchment Area study
C.   shows a good response to monoamine oxidase inhibitors
D.   is associated with major depression in 50% of patients
E.   is less likely to respond to placebo than depression

39. In child psychiatry, the EEG:

A.   in homocystinuria may show diffuse abnormalities

B.   spike and wave activity is pathognomonic of temporal lobe epilepsy

C.   spike and wave seizures are often associated with altered cardiorespiratory function

D.   during sleep is abnormal in phenylketonuria

E.   in sleep disorders such as night terrors and sleepwalking show that these usually occur on arousal from REM sleep

40. Gilles de la Tourette's syndrome:

A.   symptoms are dependent on the culture in which the sufferer was brought up

B.   usually presents initially with coprolalia

C.   may have associated gait abnormalities

D.   symptoms may be aggravated by boredom

E.   is particularly associated with psychosis

41. In Down's syndrome:

A.   the future development of children is associated with their facial appearance

B.   epileptic phenomena are exceedingly rare in infancy

C.   the peak incidence of births occurs in women aged 30-39

D.   children with the syndrome use different strategies to learn how to count compared with 'normal' children

E.   receptive language function deteriorates with age

42. Autistic disorders:

A.   have a recognised association with Gilles de la Tourette's syndrome

B.   may be related to paternal Asperger's syndrome

C.   are associated with fragile-X syndrome

D.   are often associated with right temporal lobe damage

E.   usually improve significantly with age

43. In pregnancy:

A. tricyclic antidepressants are usually teratogenic
B. lithium may cause foetal goitres to develop
C. benzodiazepines do not cross the placenta
D. barbiturates may cause withdrawal symptoms in the neonate
E. carbamazepine is absolutely contraindicated

44. Prolonged high-dose cocaine dependence is associated with:

A. restlessness
B. hypervigilance
C. convulsions
D. persecutory ideation
E. hypoacusis

45. The following are true of coma:

A. the oculovestibular response is helpful in diagnosing psychogenic coma
B. absent pupillary reflexes yet preserved reflex eye movement are typical of barbiturate-induced coma
C. coma is rarely associated with penetrating head injury in the absence of brainstem damage
D. asymmetry of the doll's head response is a sign of a focal lesion
E. lesions below the level of the pons rarely produce coma

46. Cognitive–analytic therapy:

A. was developed by Aaron Beck
B. arose out of psychotherapy sessions given to University students
C. does not involve work with the transference
D. usually lasts for a minimum of twenty-five sessions
E. usually involves reformulations given to the patient in the form of diagrams

47. In the management of epilepsy:

A. carbamazepine and sodium valproate can be given once daily because they are slowly metabolised

B. phenytoin toxicity may be precipitated by the addition of carbamazepine

C. petit mal partial seizures are best treated with ethosuximide or sodium valproate

D. carbamazepine should be avoided in patients with AV conduction disorders

E. phenobarbitone may increase serum levels of tricyclics by reducing their inactivation

48. In the management of withdrawal from opiate drugs:

A. clonidine is an alternative to methadone and is effective in reducing restlessness and autonomic symptoms

B. the supply of drugs of addiction to addicts can only be prescribed by practitioners working in drug dependency clinics

C. inpatient treatment is necessary for the first 48 hours as cardiovascular collapse may occur

D. most addicts who withdraw should no longer need methadone after three months

E. the use of MAOI drugs is contraindicated if methadone is being used as there is a danger of a hypertensive crisis

49. The following physical signs are correctly associated with the following conditions:

A. shagreen patches and tuberose sclerosis

B. wide carying angle (cubitus valgus) and Klinefelter's syndrome

C. obesity and the Lawrence–Moon–Biedl syndrome

D. cherry red spot on the macula and Niemann–Pick disease

E. ovarian dysgenesis and the Lesch–Nyhan syndrome

50. The following are true of exhibitionism:

A. the offenders are characteristically aged more than fifty
B. less than 10% of offenders are mentally retarded
C. exposure is usually a prelude to rape
D. cyproterone acetate is the treatment of choice for the recidivist offender
E. it is the most frequent parasexual activity subject to prosecution

MCQ Paper Three

Answers

1. A = T, B = F, C = T, D = F, E = F.

The fragile-X syndrome is the subject of intense research activity since it represents a fairly recent diagnosis which accounts for some 20–30% of all cases of mental retardation. The syndrome, first recognised by Martin Bell, is associated with long facies, large ears, macro-orchidism and mild-to-moderate mental retardation. One third of heterozygote females are intellectually impaired. Heterozygote females also are more prone to schizophrenia and affective disorder. Recent work has focused on the integral role of multiple CGG nucleotide arrays at the fragile site at the distal end of the X chromosome's long arm. These multiple arrays of CGG can be detected by direct DNA tests prenatally. However some 10% of pedigrees with fragile-X do not show the DNA changes at this site leading to speculation that there may be alternative nearby sites (Rousseau et al., 1991).

Hirst MC, Suthers GK, Davies KE (1992) X-linked mental retardation: the fragile-X syndrome. Hosp Update, 736-42.
Rousseau F, et al. (1991) Direct diagnosis by DNA analysis of the fragile-X syndrome of mental retardation. N Engl J Med, 325, 1673-81.

2. A = F, B = F, C = T, D = T, E = T.

Goldstein et al. (1989) looked at 332 schizophrenic men and women and found the mean age of onset for men was 24.3 years and for women 27.9 years. Angermeyer et al. (1989) found that over an eight-year follow-up period men had a greater risk of re-admission and that their admissions tended to be much longer. Boys who go on to develop schizophrenia are more likely to have antecedent defects of intellectual and social functioning than girls. On CT and MRI brain scans there is evidence that males with schizophrenia more often have structural abnormalities of neurodevelopmental origin, including things like cysts of the septum pellucidum and obstetric complications.

Angermeyer MC, Goldstein JM, Kuhn L (1989) Gender and the course of schizophrenia: differences in treated outcomes. Schizophrenia Bull, 10, 430-59.
Goldstein JM, Tsuang MT, Faraone SV (1989) Gender and schizophrenia: implications for understanding the heterogeneity of the illness. Psychiatr Res, 28, 243-53.
Lewis S (1992) Sex and schizophrenia: vive la différence. Br J Psychiatr, 161, 445-50.

3. A=F, B=T, C=F, D=T, E=T.

Morgan's (1979) definition of deliberate self-harm included both enteral and parenteral causes, and therefore included self-poisoning. The association with binge-eating and guilt in bulimia nervosa has been described by Lacey and Evans (1986). The American Psychiatric Association criteria for histrionic personality do not include deliberate self-harm. Self-harm is a feature of borderline personality disorder. Favazza (1987) likened the repetition of tension, self-cutting, and temporary relief to an addiction. Briere and Zaidi (1989) linked self-harm with childhood sexual abuse.

Briere J, Zaidi LY (1989) Sexual abuse histories and sequelae in female psychiatric emergency room patients. Am J Psychiatr, 146, 1602-6.
Favazza A (1987) Bodies under siege. Baltimore, Johns Hopkins University Press.
Lacey JH, Evans CDH (1986) The impulsivist: a multi-impulse personality disorder. Br J Addiction, 81, 641-9.
Morgan HG (1979) Death Wishes. Chichester, John Wiley.

4. **All true.**

Smoking, loneliness, lack of satisfaction with life and female sex all appeared to act as independent vulnerability factors for the genesis of depression three years later in the Liverpool Continuing Health in the Community Study. Bereavement of a close figure in the previous six months appeared to act as a trigger factor for cases of depression in the community (Green et al., 1992).

Brown and Harris (1978) performed the by-now classic community study of young working class mothers in Camberwell and reported factors associated with depression such as lack of confidant, unemployment, loss of mother before age 11 and looking after three children aged less than five years.

Brown G, Harris T (1978) Social Origins of Depression. London, Tavistock.
Green BH, Copeland JRM, Dewey ME, et al. (1992) Risk factors for depression in elderly people: a prospective study. Acta Psychiatr Scand, 86, 213-7.

5. A=T, B=F, C=T, D=T, E=F.

Blackburn et al. (1986) showed that in depression a trial of medication, or cognitive therapy (CT), or CT with amitryptyline or clomipramine, produced a relapse rate of 30%, 6% and 0% respectively; suggesting that CT has important prophylactic effects against relapse.

Social skills training helped to maintain recovery on follow-up at six and twelve months after recovery (Miller et al., 1989). In the NIMH study of 240 depressed patients imipramine was found to be superior to CT and interpersonal therapy which in turn were each superior to placebo. Imipramine was particularly effective in severely depressed patients (Elkin et al., 1989)

Blackburn IM, Eunson KM, Bishop S (1986) A two-year naturalistic follow-up of depressed patients treated with cognitive therapy, pharmacotherapy and a combination of both. J Affective Disord, 10, 67-75.
Miller IW, Norman WH, Keitner GI. (1989) Cognitive behavioural therapy of depressed inpatients: six and twelve month follow-up. Am J Psychiatr, 146, 1274-9.
Elkin I, Shea T, Watkins JT, et al. (1989) NIMH treatment of depression collaborative research program: initial outcome findings. Arch Gen Psychiatr, 46, 971-82.
Stravinsky A, Greenberg D (1992) The psychological management of depression. Acta Psychiatr Scand, 85, 407-14.

6. A = F, B = T, C = T, D = T, E = F.

In the Newcastle post-mortem study of hospitalised dementia cases the second largest group after dementia of the Alzheimer type (52%) was Lewy body type dementia (20%). In this, inclusion bodies with a core of neurofilament protein, microtubule protein, ubiquitin and tau protein are found in a variety of cortical areas. Cortical areas involved include temporal, hippocampal, cingulate, limbic and neocortical areas. In addition up to 40% of cells are lost from the substantia nigra. In Parkinson's disease up to 70% of cells in the substantia nigra must be lost before symptoms manifest. Even so, this loss of 40% of cells renders the sufferers prone to develop drug-induced extrapyramidal syndromes. Clinical features include marked fluctuations in cognitive impairment. Amnesias, apraxias and aphasias can all be seen, along with clouding of consciousness, visual and auditory hallucinations and paranoid delusions. Unlike acute organic brain syndromes clinical features may persist over weeks or months. The assessment process of patients who present in this way must rule out other physical causes, particularly cerebrovascular infarctions.

McKeith IG, Perry RH, Fairbairn AF, et al. (1992) Operational criteria for senile dementia of Lewy body type. Psychol Med, 22, 911-22.

7. A = T, B = T, C = F, D = T, E = F.

Between 1966–69 and 1978–82 there was a 150% reported increase in the incidence of anorexia nervosa leading to the speculation that cultural factors such as society's increasing concern with the cult of thinness may affect incidence rates. However, although studies, such as that from Scotland and others, have apparently shown an increase in incidence rates, there has been some criticism of methods, e.g. poor case definition according to standard criteria. It has been pointed out that in the past sufferers may not have been brought to the attention of doctors, or diagnosed if they were, and, furthermore, if they were diagnosed, put onto case registers (Szmukler, 1983). The EAT (Eating Attitudes Test) questionnaire has been shown to have good validity in a clinical setting, but, although it is of epidemiological use, it has proved less sensitive in screening general populations. Prevalence rates in some studies of eating disorders may be artificially low since anorexic people avoid answering difficult questions on eating behaviour. A reliable point-prevalence for broadly defined eating disorders in young British females is about 4–5% (King, 1989).

Cross-cultural studies have shown apparently widely differing prevalence rates which may be attributable to an actual difference in rates; or differences in concepts of what eating disorders are; or problems in translating questionnaires between cultures (Patton and King, 1991).

King MB (1989) Eating disorders in a general practice population: prevalence, characteristics and follow-up at 12–18 months. Psychol Med, suppl 14, Cambridge, Cambridge University Press.
Patton GC, King MB (1991) Epidemiological study of eating disorders: time for a change of emphasis. Psychol Med, 21, 287-91.
Szmukler GI (1983) Weight and food preoccupation in a population of English schoolgirls. In: Bargman JG (ed), Understanding Anorexia Nervosa and Bulimia Nervosa. Ohio, Ross Laboratories.

8. A = F, B = T, C = F, D = T, E = F.
The York Retreat was founded by a Quaker tea merchant, William Tuke, of the philanthropic Tuke family. The family continued to run the Retreat over several generations. William Tuke's great-grandson, Dr Daniel Hack Tuke, was an internationally renowned psychiatrist and President of the equivalent of the Royal College. Phillippe Pinel was much influenced by English psychiatry and became famous for unchaining the lunatics of the Bicêtre. The degeneration theory (which owed much to Benedict Morel) suggested that psychiatric disorders were inherited traits that worsened with successive generations; so that in the one generation neurosis might appear, which in the next generation would become depression, and in the next dementia praecox. The *Malleus Maleficarum* (or *Witches' Hammer*) was written in the sixteenth century by the Dominicans Kramer and Sprenger. The *Malleus* gave 'case histories' of various supposed witches. It helped fuel a concerted Europe-wide execution programme for the eccentric, mentally handicapped and mentally ill. Some 100,000 'witches' were destroyed. The EEG has been credited to Berger, who 'discovered' it in 1929.

9. **A = T, B = F, C = T, D = T, E = T.**
Egas Moniz was Professor of Neurology at Lisbon and was
responsible for developing leucotomy and cerebral angiography.
Cerletti used the first electrically-induced fits in catatonia in the 1930s.
Jellinek described five patterns of pathological drinking, but these are
not thought to be discrete entities. George Russell described bulimia
nervosa in 1979. Phineas Gage was a construction worker on the US
railways who survived after an explosion in which a tamping iron was
sent through his skull, damaging the frontal lobe. His subsequent
change in character was carefully described.

Russell GFM (1979) Bulimia nervosa: an ominous variant of anorexia nervosa. Psychol
Med, 9, 429.

10. **A = T, B = T, C = T, D = T, E = F.**
The Kleine–Levin syndrome is characterised by hypersomnolence,
excessive eating and disturbed sexual behaviour. The Kluver–Bucy
syndrome is associated with blunting of the emotions, agnosias,
unrestrained exploring, an oral tendency with altered eating behaviour
and hypersexuality. Medial thalamic damage may lead to a vegetative
state, and posterolateral damage may lead to abnormal sensations and
pain. Reduplicative paramnesia, which might involve someone
maintaining that they are simultaneously at home and in the hospital,
is attributable to a lesion of the parietal lobe.

11. **All false.**
Numerical ability is relatively spared in Pick's disease, which
predominantly affects the frontal and temporal lobes, unlike
Alzheimer's which initially affects parietal and medial temporal lobes.
Status spongiosus is characteristic of Creutzfeldt–Jakob disease.
Ventricular dilatation out of proportion to sulcal atrophy is a feature
of normal pressure hydrocephalus.

12. **All true.**
Response prevention is used to reduce obsessional rituals, and to be
effective must be self-imposed. Exposure reduces both obsessional
rituals and associated anxiety (Foa et al., 1980) In cue exposure the
link between the stimulus (that triggers the unwanted behaviour) and
the behaviour itself is weakened by allowing the stimulus to continue
and preventing the usual response. Habit reversal focuses on providing
an alternative behaviour that is incompatible with the unwanted

behaviour. Stimulus control focuses on modifying or avoiding the stimuli that initiate unwanted behaviours, for instance if the salesman's daily walk to work takes him past the supermarket where he can buy his morning alcohol, an alternative route might be taken. Introducing a delay mechanism between stimulus and response aims to hasten extinguishment of the behaviour. An example of such a delay is increasing the length of time between an anorexic's meal and her vomiting.

Foa EB, Steketee G, Milby JB (1980) Differential effects of exposure and response prevention in obsessive-compulsive washers. J Consult Clin Psychol, 48, 71-9.

13. A = T, B = T, C = T, D = F, E = F.

Jerome Frank and others have emphasised the importance of the expectations of improvement that the patient brings with him or her into the group, and these expectations are heightened when he or she sees others in the group improving (Frank, 1961). Universality comes into play when patients learn that others in the group may have had very similar experiences and feelings. Vicarious learning is where the patient benefits from other members' therapy experiences or models new future behaviours on the therapist or other patients. Resistance occurs in the context of analytic therapies, but is not one of the most positive therapeutic factors in group work. Enmeshment describes a particular structural problem in families in family therapy.

Frank JD (1961) Persuasion and Healing. Baltimore, Johns Hopkins Press.

14. A = T, B = T, C = F, D = T, E = F.

Systems theory was described by von Bertalaffny in 1973. Homeostasis is the mechanism where a system (family) in steady state will compensate for any change, or resist attempts to impose or create change. Systems like families have subsystems (e.g. marital and sibling). In families causality is circular not linear and feedback loops may operate.

von Bertalaffny L (1973) General Systems Theory. Foundations, Development, Applications. New York, George Braziller.

15. A = F, B = T, C = T, D = T, E = F.

The injection of sodium amytal (called the WADA technique) into one carotid artery will anaesthetize one hemisphere, so that testing can be performed on the opposite hemisphere. However the procedure is not without risk.

16. A = T, B = T, C = F, D = F, E = T.

Total institutions like prisons, special hospitals, asylums and monasteries have all-encompassing tendencies. They break down the normal separations that we all enjoy between work, play and sleep, in that all activities are under the same authority in the same place. All activities are tightly scheduled and occur in the name of some rational plan according to the aims of the institution. There is a split between a large managed group (inmates/patients) and a small supervisory group (prison officers/nurses). Communication between inmates to higher staff levels (e.g. patients to doctors) is controlled (e.g. by nurses).

Goffman E (1961) Asylums. Harmondsworth, Penguin.

17. A = T, B = T, C = F, D = T, E = T.

Toffler in 1970 described culture shock, which happens when people are plunged, inadequately prepared, into an alien culture. Rack (1986) suggested that there were three types of migrant: a gastarbeiter, or guest worker, who intends to return; an exile who migrates after political upheaval or natural disaster; and the settler who migrates with positive expectations. Refugees would count as 'exiles' in Rack's classification. Refugees have a particularly high psychiatric morbidity because of prior trauma which may cause post-traumatic stress disorder, or trigger affective illness or schizophrenia. Acculturation (Herz, 1988) is the adaptive coping process affecting immigrants. Hemsi in 1967 reported a study where the incidence of schizophrenia in West Indian immigrants was almost five times higher than in British-born black people. Explanations for this have been extensively discussed (Cochrane and Bal, 1977).

Cochrane R, Bal SS (1977) Migration and schizophrenia: an examination of five hypotheses. Soc Psychiatr. 22, 181-91.
Herz DG (1988) Identity, lost and found: patterns of migration and psychological and psychosocial adjustment of migrants. Acta Psychiatr Scand, 78 (Suppl 344) 159-65.
Rack PH (1986) Migration and mental illness. In: Cox JL (ed), Transcultural Psychiatry. London, Croom Helm.

18. A=T, B=T, C=T, D=F, E=F.

Successful families provide a setting in which members can fulfil their potential. They provide the initial model for socialisation which can be transferred to the outside world. Parents provide a model for future sexual identity, but there must also be boundaries demarcating the parents from the children, which the children can accept, and where the leadership role of the parents is respected.

Bentovim A (1986) Family therapy. In: Bloch S (ed), Introduction to the Psychotherapies. Oxford, Oxford Medical Publications.
Henderson AS (1988) Social treatments and preventive strategies. In: An Introduction to Social Psychiatry. Oxford, Oxford Medical Publications.

19. A=F, B=T, C=F, D=T, E=F.

All the diagnoses A–E are categories in disorders of psychological development. Specific speech articulation disorder is in disorders of speech and language. Childhood autism is an example of pervasive developmental disorder, as is Rett's syndrome.

20. All true.

Lishman WA (1987) Organic Psychiatry, 2nd Edn. London, Blackwells.

21. A=T, B=F, C=F, D=F, E=T.

The Wechsler Adult Intelligence Scale (WAIS) has 11 sub-tests divided between verbal and performance tests. Verbal sub-tests include information, comprehension, arithmetic, similarities, digit span, and vocabulary. Performance sub-tests include digit symbol, picture completion, block design, picture arrangement, and object assembly, The WAIS gives an intelligence quotient, and has a role in identifying brain damage by showing discrepancies between verbal and performance IQs. The perceptual maze test (1955) can detect brain damage caused by quite small focal lesions.

Wechsler D (1958) The Measurement and Appraisal of Adult Intelligence, 4th Edn. Baltimore, Williams and Wilkins.

22. A=F, B=F, C=T, D=T, E=T.

Voluntary patient status was a concept introduced in the 1930s. Group therapy began with groups of tuberculosis patients and lectures from their doctor, Dr Pratt, in 1905.

23. A=F, B=F, C=T, D=T, E=F.

Erectile impotence occurs in 1.9% of 40-year-olds (Kinsey et al., 1948). In Frank's 1978 self-report survey of 100 couples, 77% of wives and 50% of husbands had some sexual problems. 12% of psychiatric clinic attenders report sexual problems and marital difficulties (Swan and Wilson, 1979). Erectile dysfunction occurs in 7–10% of males, compared with 20–40% for premature ejaculation.

Frank E, Anderson C, Kupfer DJ (1976) Profiles of couples seeking sex therapy and marital therapy. Am J Psychiatr, 133, 559-62.
Kinsey AC, Pomeroy WB, Martin CE (1948) Sexual Behaviour in the Human Male. Phildelphia, Saunders.
Swan M, Wilson LJ (1979) Sexual and marital problems in a psychiatric out-patient population. Br J Psychiatr, 135, 310-14.
Thornes B, Collard J (1979) Who Divorces? London, Routledge and Kegan Paul.

24. A=F, B=F, C=F, D=F, E=T.

An anatomically correct doll would be useful in an interview with a younger child; instead, art and drawing materials might be used, including more detailed anatomical drawing. By the age of 10 or 12, a child can be as proficent at recall as an adult. In an initial investigative interview there is 'no place' for education or lectures as to what the boundaries should be between adults and children. The aim is to find out if anything inappropriate has happened and what exactly that was. Enabling questions can be used with care to facilitate a difficult interview, but the use of the child's own language is important and the introduction of leading questions is to be avoided. Gaze fixation should be limited, but embarrassment and the appearance of embarrassment avoided.

Jones DPH, McQuiston MG (1988) Interviewing the Sexually Abused Child. London, Gaskell.

25. A=T, B=F, C=T, D=F, E=T.

Winnicott saw interpretation in analytic treatment as a sophisticated extension of infant care, and therefore more than just an echo of the mother–infant relationship. Before a child can communicate using language, the mother has a 'magical understanding' of her child's needs. So, the infant's primary capacity for communication pre-dates the acquisition of language. Winnicott was critical of silent analysts who pretend to understand everthing, becoming a seductive impostor of the originally omnipotent mother. The silent analyst tries to emulate the 'magical understanding' of the mother. The therapist should voice trial interpretations, but the interpretation is only good to the patient if it can be owned by them, exemplified by Winnicott's paradoxical statement: 'the statement must be found in order to be created.'

Winnicott D (1986) Holding and Interpretation: Fragment of an Analysis. London, Hogarth Press.
Winnicott D (1971) Therapeutic Consultation in Child Psychiatry. London, Hogarth Press.

BG

26. A = T, B = T, C = T, D = F, E = T.

Frontal lobe tumours commonly present with symptoms of confusion, personality change and dementia. Psychiatric symptoms were the first to appear in anteriorly placed frontal lobe tumours in over one-third of cases. A greater frequency of mental abnormality has been described in patients with gliomas than in those with meningiomas. This is probably related to the greater rate of growth of the former. Pre-motor damage leads to incontinence, aphasia, akinesia, mutism and apraxia. Depression is infrequent and intracranial tumours are rare in patients with affective disorder in the absence of neurological signs.

Ron MA (1989) Psychiatric manifestations of frontal lobe tumours. Br J Psychiatr, 155, 735-8.

27. A = T, B = F, C = T, D = T, E = T.

There is evidence that bilateral ECT is more effective that unilateral possibly since fit induction is more reliable. Studies of ECT efficacy have consistently demonstrated its superiority over MAOIs. MAOIs often appear to be most effective in patients with reversed functional shift but, as tricyclics are also effective and safer, irreversible MAOIs remain second choice. A number of trials have demonstrated the superiority of tricyclics over placebo in patients with mild-to-moderate depression. People with very mild depression (Hamilton Rating Scale < 13) showed no difference between tricyclics and placebo. Most of the studies of cognitive therapy have been done in patients with mild-to-moderate depression and suggest that in this group cognitive therapy is as effective as drug therapy.

Paykel E (1989) Features of depression. Br J Psychiatr, 155, 754-63.

28. A = F, B = T, C = T, D = F, E = F.

Loss of personal (episodic) memories is more suggestive of an organic lesion and its return marks the end of post-traumatic amnesia. Loss of personal identity is more suggestive of psychogenic amnesia. Forgetfulness tends to persist despite compensation.

(1987) Amnesia: organic and psychogenic. Br Med J, 150, 428-42.

29. A = F, B = T, C = F, D = T, E = T.

Complex partial seizures (CPS) are associated with impairment of consciousness and loss of consciousness can occur from the outset. Tumours are found in 10–15% of adults presenting with CPS. Speech automatisms (bursts of incorrect, inappropriate speech) suggest the right temporal lobe. Forced thinking is a compulsion to think on certain topics e.g. death.

30. A = T, B = T, C = F, D = F, E = T.

Writer's cramp is one of the occupational cramps which causes an impairment of some educated motor skill due to motor spasm. The aetiology is unclear. Writer's cramp is more common in men. The onset is in the third and fourth decades. In contrast to dystonic writer's cramp, in simple writer's cramp the symptoms generally only appear on writing. The dystonic form may rarely be associated with a torsion dystonia and torticollis. Writer's cramp tends to run a fluctuating course but is chronically progressive in the majority of cases. Finger movements tend to be jerky and inco-ordinated and tremor may be prominent.

Lishman WA (1987) Organic Psychiatry, 2nd Edn. London, Blackwell.
Sheehy MP, Marsden CD (1982) Writer's cramp – a focal dystonia. Brain, 105, 461-80.

31. A = T, B = F, C = F, D = F, E = F.

The incidence range is 1 per 10,000 to 1 per 20,000 live births. PKU is inherited in an autosomal recessive fashion. It is screened for using the Guthrie test only after several days on milk feeds. Seizures occur in approximately 25% of cases. Infants with PKU have similar minimal requirements of phenylalanine to normal children. Too severe a restriction can lead to tissue breakdown and rising levels of phenylalanine.

32. A=T, B=F, C=T, D=F, E=F.

Episodic dyscontrol syndrome (Bach-y-Rita et al., 1971) is characterised by uncontrollable aggression on minimal provocation. It is associated with non-specific EEG abnormalities including temporal lobe spikes. It tends to decline in only 40% in the fourth decade. Auras preceding the outbursts take the form of hyperacusis, visual illusions, numbness and nausea. Alcohol and chlordiazepoxide both increase liability to attacks. Some reports have suggested the use of lithium or propranolol in controlling outbursts. No specific category of 'episodic dyscontrol' appears in ICD-10 or DSM-III-R. DSM-III-R does contain a category, '312.34 Intermittent explosive disorder', which involves 'several discrete episodes of loss of control of aggresive impulses resulting in serious assaultive acts or destruction of property. These episodes occur 'out or proportion to any precipitating psychosocial stressors'. In ICD-10 intermittent explosive disorder is subsumed under 'F63.8 Other habit and impulse disorders'.

Bach-y-Rita G, et al. (1971) Episodic dyscontrol: a study of 130 violent patients. Am J Psychiatr, 127, 1473-8.

33. A=F, B=T, C=T, D=T, E=F.

There has been little development in the psychological management of erectile impotence in the last decade. Psychological treatment appears to have more effect on marital satisfaction than on sexual functioning. Intracavernosal injection of papaverine causes a pharmacologically induced erection and also leads to an improvement in spontaneous erectile function, possibly by decreasing anxiety and increasing confidence. Suction devices produce erections adequate for penetration but not a full erection, the penis tending to hang rather than stand up. Headache in the partner has been described as a result of transvaginal absorption of the topical nitroglycerine. This problem could be overcome by the wearing of a condom. Priapism responds to local injection of an α-adrenergic agonist e.g. phenylephrine.

Gregoire A (1992) New treatments for erectile impotence. Br J Psychiatr, 160, 315-26.

34. A=T, B=F, C=F, D=F, E=T.

'Shopping around' has been described by Professor Bicknell in families fixated at the denial stage. 'Bargaining' with professionals occurs before acceptance. 'Ego-centred work/family-centred work' follows acceptance and involves appropriate help-seeking behaviour. The 'fantasy' stage of acceptance helps families to cope with their plight and should be allowed to run its course. 'Infantilisation' is characterised by acceptance of the child with a handicap (the handicapped adult being far less accepted).

Bicknell J (1983) The psychopathology of handicap. Br J Med Psychol, 56, 167-78.

35. A = T, B = T, C = T, D = F, E = T.

The EEG in Huntington's disease characteristically shows poorly developed or complete loss of alpha rhythms. The record may flatten as the disease progresses. Atrophy of the caudate and putamen occur, but other nuclei tend to be spared. Memory impairment can usually be demonstrated within a year of onset of the chorea, but is rarely severe and is relatively less afected than other cognitive functions. Cognitive decline in the absence of language disorder is characteristic of Huntington's disease and suggests a sub-cortical origin for the dementia. Distractibility is a marked, characteristic feature.

36. A = F, B = T, C = F, D = F, E = F.

Mood alteration is an immediate and prominent effect of opiate use. Patients may feel drowsy or describe a dream-like state, but, unlike alcohol, marked changes in consciousness are not a prominent feature. The withdrawal syndrome is typified by insomnia, agitation, myalgia, abdominal pain, rhinorrhoea, diarrhoea, dilated pupils, tachycardia and temperature disturbance. Opiate withdrawal begins within six hours and peaks at 36 hours. Flashbacks occur with LSD and cannabis. Opiates are not hallucinogenic and paranoid psychosis does not generally occur.

37. A = F, B = T, C = T, D = T, E = F.

60–70% of depressed patients respond to the first antidepressant drug and a further 10–15% respond to the use of an alternative drug or ECT. Approximately 20% of patients fail to respond to initial treatment. Poor prognosis has been related to the duration of the illness prior to beginning treatment, delusional depression, few life events prior to the depression and associated physical illness. Chronicity and high neuroticism also predict poor outcome. Lithium augmentation is associated with a 50% increase in response rate. The response rate of delusional depression to tricyclics in studies varies from 30–40%. The addition of an antipsychotic increases the response rate to 78%.

Duggan CF, et al. (1990) Does personality predict long-term outcome in depression? Br J Psychiatr, 157, 19-24.

Goodwin G (1990) Drug treatment of depression: what if tricyclics don't work? In: Dilemmas and Difficulties in the Management of Psychiatric Patients. Oxford, Oxford Medical Publications.

Leonard BE (1988) Therapy-resistant depression. Br J Psychiatr, 152, 453-9.

Magri (1988) Clinical correlates of ECT resistant depression in the elderly. J Clin Psychiatr, 49, 405-7.

Katona CLE (1989) Lithium augmentation in refractory depression. Psychiatr Devel, 2, 153-71

38. A=F, B=T, C=F, D=F, E=T.

The sex distribution for obsessive–compulsive disorder (OCD) for women:men is about 1–1.5 : 1. Unlike anxiety states, OCD shows a poor response to conventional anxiolytics. In the ECA one-third of patients with OCD also fulfilled the criteria for major depression. A placebo response of 5% has been shown in OCD whereas depression enjoys a 30% placebo response rate.

AO'H

39. A=T, B=F, C=T, D=T, E=F.

Diffuse abnormalities on the EEG are shown in homocystinuria, porphyria and Hartnup disease amongst others. Spike and wave activity may occur in children with or without epilepsy. Sleep disorders such as night terrors and somnambulism usually occur on arousal from stage IV or non-REM sleep.

Fenwick P (1985) The EEG. In: Rutter M, Hersov L (eds), Child and Adolescent Psychiatry. Oxford, Blackwell, 280-303.

40. A=F, B=F, C=T, D=T, E=F.

Symptoms of Tourette's syndrome are largely independent of culture. Motor tics of the head are the initial presentation at a mean age of seven years. Vocal tics may start around the age of eleven, and coprolalia (which occurs in 30% of patients) begins around the age of thirteen. Tourette's syndrome is not asssociated with psychosis, but is associated with depression, habit disorders, enuresis, and obsessional disorders.

Robertson MM (1989) The Gilles de la Tourette syndrome: the current status. Br J Psychiatr, 154, 147-69.

41. A = F, B = F, C = F, D = F, E = T.

The 'severity' of facial stigmata of Down's syndrome do not appear to affect development in terms of intelligence quotient, self-sufficiency, and family functioning. Seizures occur in about 7% of people with Down's. Various authors comment on the frequency of infantile spasms. The peak incidence of Down's births is in women aged 20-29. Children with Down's use the same strategies to learn counting as younger children without Down's syndrome. Early indicators of dementia in people with Down's syndrome include impairment of receptive language.

Cunningham C, et al. (1991) Is the appearance of children with Down's syndreom associated with their development and social functioning? Devel Med Child Neurol, 33, 285-95.
Safstrom CE, et al. (1991) Seizures in children with Down's syndrome : aetiology, characteristics and outcome. Devel Med Child Neurol, 33, 191-200.
Young EC, Kramer BM (1991) Characteristics of age-related language decline in adults with Down's syndrome. Ment Retard 29, 75-9.

42. A = T, B = T, C = T, D = F, E = F.

24% of the parents of autistic children have anxiety disorders prior to the birth of the autistic child. 12% of fathers have Asperger's. The conversational language of parents of autistic children often has autistiform elements. Autistic features have developed in children and an adult with left (dominant) temporal lobe abnormalities, but there is no persistent link to right temporal lobe damage. The future course of autistic disorders can be predicted largely from childhood psychometric testing. Follow-up of individuals suggests little overall shift in ability levels.

Freeman BJ, et al. (1991) The stability of cognitive and behavioural parameters in autism: a twelve year prospective study. J Am Acad Child Adolesc Psychiatr, 30, 479-82.
Gillberg C, Gillberg IC, Steffenburg S (1992) Siblings and parents of children with autism: a controlled population-based study. Devel Med Child Neurol, 34, 389-98.
Landa R, et al. (1992) Social language use in parents of autistic individuals. Psychol Med, 22, 245-54.

43. A = F, B = T, C = F, D = T, E = F.

Tricyclic antidepressants are associated with case reports of difficulty in late pregnancy – CNS depression, respiratory acidosis, and convulsions. Benzodiazepines do cross the placenta and because the foetal liver metabolism is minimal benzodiazepines are concentrated in foetal tissues.

44. A = T, B = T, C = T, D = T, E = F.

BG

45. A = T, B = F, C = T, D = F, E = T.

The oculovestibular response is abnormal in organic coma, a tonic response occurs in cortical lesions, an assymetrical response suggests a focal brain stem lesion or a drug-induced coma. Absence of the response occurs in profound brain stem disturbance or drug overdose coma. Nystagmus occurs in normally alert individual and should suggest psychogenic coma. Preservation of pupillary reflexes with loss of reflex eye movement in a coma patient suggests a drug-induced coma. Assymetrical oculocephalic response (DHR) is a sign of a brain stem lesion but can occur in a drug-induced coma.

46. A = F, B = T, C = F, D = F, E = T.

Cognitive–analytic therapy (CAT) derives from the work of Anthony Ryle, who was a director of Sussex University's Health Service until 1979 and later became a consultant psychotherapist. Beck developed cognitive therapy (1976). Recent CAT studies have focused on patients being usefully given between 12 and 16 sessions of CAT rather than 'a minimum of twenty-five'. The therapy work uses fairly classical concepts such as transference, interpretations and dream work associated with newer tools such as target problems, target problem procedures and sequential diagrammatic reformulations. In the latter the patient and therapist work out typical sequences of behaviour that the patient performs and often relates these to parental attributes.

Beck AT (1976) Cognitive Therapy and the Emotional Disorders. New York, International Universities Press.
Ryle A (1991) Cognitive–analytic Therapy: Active Participation in Change. Chichester, John Wiley.

47. A = F, B = T, C = T, D = T, E = F.

Carbamazepine and sodium valproate need to be given several times daily as they are rapidly metabolised in contrast to phenytoin and phenobarbitone which are prescribed once daily. Carbamazepine displaces phenytoin from plasma proteins increasing the unbound form and increasing the risk of toxicity. Carbamazepine should be avoided in AV conduction disorders and porphyria. By inducing liver enzymes carbamazepine reduces the serum levels of psychotropic drugs and itself. Phenobarbitone increases liver hydroxylase production and this may increase tricyclic metabolism and decrease serum level for a given dose.

Crammer and Hare. The Use of Drugs in Psychiatry, 3rd Edn. London, Gaskell.

48. A=T, B=F, C=F, D=F, E=T.

Clonidine is a centrally acting α_2-adrenergic agonist and can be used as an alternative to methadone for opiate withdrawal. Simultaneous prescription is safe. It suppresses the autonomic disturbance effectively. The legal supply of drugs of addiction is only possible through practitioners licensed by the Home Office and the prescription must be carefully written in words and figures. Some districts may limit prescription to doctors at drug dependency clinics. Many addicts remain on a low dose of methadone indefinitely which is considered preferable to injecting street heroin. As methadone is a synthetic opioid it interacts with MAOI and a hypertensive crisis may occur.

49. A=T, B=F, C=T, D=T, E=F.

Adenoma sebaceum, cafe-au-lait spots and shagreen patches occur in tuberose sclerosis. A wide carrying angle is characteristic of Turner's syndrome (XO). Obesity, hypogonadism, retinitis pigmentosa, polydactyly, diabetes mellitus and severe handicap typify Lawrence–Moon–Biedl syndrome. Lesch–Nyhan syndrome is X-linked.

50. A=F, B=T, C=F, D=F, E=T.

Exposure is the deliberate exposure of the genitalia by a man in the presence of an unwilling woman, where the man has no intention of progression to sexual intercourse. The majority of offenders are young men aged 15–25 years. Only 5% have mental retardation. 20% of offenders are 'sociopathic' and expose an erection for sadistic pleasure; their prognosis is worse. Behavioural techniques including aversive therapy and covert sensitisation together with group therapy are the preferred treatments. Cyproterone acetate has a limited role.

Bancroft J (1989) Human Sexuality and its Problems. Edinbirgh, Churchill Livingstone.

AO'H

Short Answer Questions

GENERAL APPROACH

The MCQ exam can seem endless in terms of time. The last half-an-hour or so of the MCQ exam is often filled with a mixture of anxiety, guilt and boredom. Whereas multiple choice exams often seem over-generously timed, the Royal College SAQ exam demands that you work at a very fast pace to answer all the questions. It is not uncommon for candidates to run out of time. The SAQ exam therefore requires a change of strategy. It is important to remember that each part of the exam has a fixed set of marks to aim for (and these are specified to help you). Each question has twenty marks allotted to it and these are often broken down into sections. This has the benefit to the College that answers are discrete, short and easily marked. It has the advantage to the candidate that he or she can see exactly where to go to collect most marks. It makes no sense to concentrate on lengthy answers to elements that will yield two marks and to skimp on answers to sections worth ten marks. It is also important to remember that negative marking is not employed. This means that sometimes guessing may well yield extra marks.

You will need to strike a balance between brevity and over-inclusive verbosity. The former may not convince the examiner that you know enough to award you the marks and the latter irritates the examiner to screams. You must therefore write sufficient for the examiner to be in no doubt that you know what you are writing about and yet avoid an essay-style construction. Short sentences would be ideal, but because time is pressed in this exam, two- or three-word points may be all that is possible. If nothing else, the SAQ exam experience should teach you how to communicate complicated ideas as simply as possible. Bear in mind that you will lose marks for an ill-constructed or ambiguous answer. Untidy answers that cannot be deciphered similarly lose marks for you. So, think carefully about the structure of your answer before you begin, be concise, and write legibly.

Below is a full SAQ exam. It is most important that you try this under exam conditions to get a feel of just how pressed the SAQ exam is and so that you can learn an efficient style. The answers that follow this section are necessarily brief, and can be used as pointers for further reading.

Short Answer Questions
(MRCPsych Part II)
One-and-a-half hours
20 questions

QUESTIONS

1. List 5 different mechanisms by which genetic abnormalities may be
transmitted. *(10 marks)*
Give an example of each mechanism which may cause mental
handicap. *(10 marks)*

2. After childbirth what is the risk of occurrence of
    (a) postpartum blues?
    (b) puerperal depression?
    (c) puerperal psychosis? *(6 marks)*
Give three factors which may predispose to puerperal psychosis.
(6 marks)
Describe four vulnerability factors for depression according to the
work of Brown and Harris (1978).
(8 marks)

3. (a) List 5 biochemical abnormalities found in anorexia nervosa.
(5 marks)
    (b) List 5 medical complications of anorexia nervosa.
(5 marks)
    (c) Describe the main features and epidemiology of bulimia
nervosa. *(10 marks)*

4. (a) List the seven features of the alcohol dependence syndrome as
described by Edwards and Gross.
(14 marks)
    (b) List three neuropathological features in Korsakoff's psychosis
and three organic syndromes affecting the central nervous
system caused by alcohol (other than the Wernicke–Korsakoff
syndrome).
(6 marks)

5. (a) Describe the four basic types of cognitive distortions which may be addressed by cognitive therapy.

(8 marks)

(b) List twelve curative factors in group therapy as described by Yalom. *(12 marks)*

6. Write short notes on the neuroleptic malignant syndrome with regard to aetiology *(4 marks)*, clinical features *(8 marks)* and management *(8 marks)*.

7. (a) List five causes of foetal malformations (other than alcohol or prescribed drugs).

(5 marks)

(b) List features of the foetal alcohol syndrome.

(7 marks)

(c) What effects on the foetus and neonate may be produced by lithium taken by the mother during pregnancy and in the post-natal period?

(8 marks)

8. Give ten clinical features of delirium tremens.

(10 marks)

Describe the management of delirium tremens.

(10 marks)

9. Compare and contrast pseudobulbar palsy and bulbar palsy.

(20 marks)

10. (a) Define the five axes used in DSM-III-R.

(10 marks)

(b) Describe three different types of study which support the theory that a genetic factor is implicated in the aetiology of schizophrenia.

(6 marks)

(c) Briefly describe the findings of Vaughn and Leff (1976) with regard to the role of environment and schizophrenia.

(4 marks)

11. (a)   Give four endocrine conditions important in the aetiology of depression.

(8 marks)

    (b)   Give three pieces of evidence in favour of the monoamine theory of depression.

(6 marks)

    (c)   Give six foodstuffs which may interact with phenelzine.

(6 marks)

12. What are risk factors for suicide in people with schizophrenia?

(6 marks)

What factors predict poor outcome in schizophrenia?

(12 marks)

13. (a)   Define the levels of alcohol consumption considered safe and hazardous in males and females as described by the Royal College of Psychiatrists in 1986.

(12 marks)

    (b)   Describe the CAGE alcohol screening questions.

(8 marks)

14. Compare and contrast the contributions of social learning theory and Freudian psychoanalytic theory to the understanding of motivational factors in aggression.

(20 marks)

15. Write short notes on the following aspects of human communications theory:

    (a)   Pragmatics   *(2 marks)*
    (b)   Analogic and digital communication   *(8 marks)*
    (c)   Symmetrical and complementary interaction   *(8 marks)*
    (d)   Semantics   *(2 marks)*

16. (a)   List four possible neurological complications of phenothiazine medication.

(8 marks)

    (b)   Discuss the management of three of these complications.

(12 marks)

17. List 10 priorities in the management of a suicidal patient.

(20 marks)

18. (a) Explain the concept of reliability of a research instrument and give four examples of different forms of reliability.

(10 marks)

(b) List five difficulties that should be taken into account when planning psychotherapy research.

(10 marks)

19. (a) List five causes of transient global amnesia.

(5 marks)

(b) Give five causes of dementia with some reversibility.

(5 marks)

(c) Describe five neuropathological findings in boxers' brains at post-mortem.

(10 marks)

20. List six different types of intracranial tumour.

(6 marks)

What are the characteristic focal signs and symptoms of tumours in the:

(a) frontal lobe, *(6 marks)*
(b) temporal lobe, *(4 marks)*
(c) corpus callosum? *(4 marks)*

ANSWERS

1.

Dominant gene: Tuberous sclerosis
Recessive gene (errors of metabolism): Phenylketonuria
Extra chromosome (autosome): Down's (21), Edward's (18), Patau (13–15)
Deleted chromosome (autosome): 'cri du chat' (chromosome No. 5)
Extra sex chromosome: XXY Klinefelter's, 'XXX superfemale'
Deleted sex chromosome: XO Turner's
Sex-linked recessive: Hunters, Lesch–Nyhan   PDM

2.

(a)   0.2%

(b)   10:15%

(c)   50%
        3 from: Primigravida, unmarried, history of manic depression, history
        of schizophrenia, perinatal death, Caesarian section

        Not working outside home, unsupportive partner, 3 or more children
        under 15 at home, loss of mother before age 11
                                                               PDM

3.

(a) 5 from

Leucopenia	Decreased gonadotrophins
Lymphocytosis	Decreased gonadal steroids
Alkalosis	Increased growth hormone
Decreased potassium	Decreased T3
Decreased glucose	Increased cortisol
Increased cholesterol	Hypercarotenaemia
Increased amylase	

(b) 5 from

Bradycardia	Decreased growth
Hypotension	Hypothermia
Cardiac arrhythmias	Salivary gland enlargement
Oedema	Impaired gastric emptying
Cardiac failure	Acute gastric dilatation

Fits

Amenorrhoea

Osteoporosis and
  pathological fractures

Acute pancreatitis

Tetany

Superior mesenteric artery syndrome

Constipation

Dehydration

Hypoglycaemia

Enamel erosion

Caries

(c) *Features*

Loss of control over eating with irresistible cravings for food

High calorie binges, secretly and with insight

Purging/vomiting/dieting/appetite suppressant drugs/diuretics as compensation

Preoccupation with weight and body shape

At least two binges weekly for at least three months (DSM-III-R)

Epidemiology:

Mostly females

Middle and upper socioeconomic classes (about 1% prevalence)

Often preceded by anorexia nervosa

Adolescence (late) or early adulthood

Family history of obesity, depression, and/or alcoholism

PDM

4.

(a)   Stereotyped drinking patterns

Predominance of drink-seeking behaviour

Increased alcohol tolerance

Repeated withdrawal symptoms

Relief or avoidance of withdrawal symptoms by further drinking

Subjective compulsion to drink

Reinstatement after abstinence

(b)   Three neuropathological findings in the Wernicke–Korsakoff syndrome:

Wernicke's encephalopathy:

lesions of walls of third ventricle,

periaqueductal region,

floor of fourth ventricle,

certain thalamic nuclei,

mamillary bodies,

terminal parts of the fornices,

brain stem and parts of the cerebellum

Korsakoff state:
    supratentorial atrophy
    sulcal and convolutional atrophy
    ventricular dilatation

Three other organic CNS problems secondary to alcohol excess:
    Marchiafava–Bignami disease
    central pontine myelinosis
    ambylopia
    cerebellar degeneration.

PDM/BG

5.

(a)   Arbitrary inference, selective abstraction, over-generalisation, minimisation and magnification.

(b)   Catharsis, insight, group cohesiveness, interpersonal learning, existential awareness, universality, altruism, installation of hope, development of socialising techniques, guidance, imitative behaviour, corrective recapititulation of the family group.

PDM

6.

Neuroleptic malignant syndrome

Aetiology
Unclear. Idiosyncratic reaction to certain drugs including neuroleptics such as haloperidol and depot fluphenazine. Dopamine blockade of the basal ganglia or hypothalamus has been implicated. May occur with 'atypical' agents such as lithium. May be precipitated by dehydration. Organic brain disease may predispose. Possibly more common in males.

Clinical features
Features may develop days or weeks after introduction of treatment. Hyperthermia, muscular rigidity (with dystonia, opisthotonus and sometimes dysphagia as well), akinesia, clouded consciousness, autonomic changes (hypertension, tachycardia, hyperventilation, sialorrhoea, sweating and pallor). Fluctuating level of consciousness. Raised white cell count, raised muscle CPK, abnormal liver function tests, elevated potassium, slow waves on EEG. High mortality.

Management

Withdrawal of medication. Supportive and symptomatic treatment, e.g. ventilatory support in severe cases where respiratory function is compromised, or re-hydration, or antibiotics for superimposed chest infection. In some patients dantrolene sodium, peripheral muscle relaxants and/or bromocriptine may be useful. ECT has been rarely advocated.

AO'H

7.

(a) (i) Radiation: ionising radiation (causes microcephaly and brain damage in first mid-trimester)

(ii) Maternal disease: diabetes mellitus (raises incidence of abnormalities from 2% to 6%; ? due to maternal disease or external insulin)

(iii) Infection: toxoplasmosis (intrauterine growth retardation, microcephaly, hydrocephaly, microphthalmia), rubella (microcephaly, patent ductus arteriosus, hepatosplenomegaly, encephalitis, cataracts and more)

(iv) Diet/environmental factors:

folic acid deficiency

excess intake of vitamins A or D

pollution e.g. dioxins

(v) Genetic: trisomy 13 or 18 (Edwards' syndrome: mental retardation, long, narrow skull, congenital heart disease, low-set ears, hare lip) and others, e.g. achondroplasia.

(b) Disorders in some of the offspring of persistently heavy drinkers:

intrauterine growth retardation

failure to thrive

short stature and developmental delay

mild-to-moderate mental retardation with language delay

characteristic facies: microcephaly, thin upper lip, small philtrum, microphthalmia, prominent forehead and maxillary hypoplasia

hyperactivity with poor muscle tone

also cleft palate, cardiac abnormalities and gait abnormalities have been described.

(c) Lithium crosses the placental barrier and during pregnancy may produce cardiac abnormalities e.g. Ebstein's anomaly (components of tricuspid valve displaced into the right ventricle leading to congestive heart failure and cyanosis). Such cardiovascular malformations may occur in about 10% of babies born to mothers on lithium in the first trimester. Other teratogenic effects may occur.

Foetal hypothyroidism and goitre may arise from use in later pregnancy. If lithium has to be used during late pregnancy and babies are born with a low serum lithium level they may have a flaccid appearance which improves spontaneously (hypotonia).

If babies are born with a high lithium level, they may require fluid therapy in the neonatal period to avert renal damage in the neonate. However use during late pregnancy increases risk of foetal death, cyanosis, bradycardia and arrhythmia in the neonate even when lithium within therapeutic range in the mother (although most risk when diuretics or restricted salt intake used in mother).

Lithium is secreted in breast milk (at 30–100% of maternal serum concentration) and therefore bottle-feeding is recommended in the infants of mothers on lithium.

AO'H/BG

8.

10 from:

Coarse tremor, disorientation, agitation, tachycardia, sweating, pyrexia, vivid hallucinosis: visual, auditory or somatic, (Lilliputian hallucinations are classical). Insomnia. Fleeting persecutory delusions. Fluctuating level of consciousness. Slurred speech. Suggestibility. Labile affect. Dehydration. Hypertension. Cardiovascular collapse. Arrhythmias. Susceptibility to infection or head trauma. Occasional hyperthermia. Seizures. Hypoglycaemia. Hypophosphataemia. Hypomagnesemia. Develops 2nd to 5th day after stopping alcohol (although in 5% of cases onset may be after one week or so of abstinence). May persist for 3–7 days. 5–15% mortality.

Management

hospitalise onto medical ward

fluid replacement: orally or i.v.

thiamine and multivitamin injections (before carbohydrates)

chlormethiazole or diazepam to control withdrawal features, sedate and raise epileptic threshold

frequent monitoring of physical state to detect concurrent infections or head injury

ECG, skull or chest X-rays may be necessary

nurse in light, ground-floor room

relevant blood investigations (minimum full blood count, urea and electrolytes, glucose) and electrolyte replacement. AO'H

9.

Both pseudobulbar palsy (PBP) and bulbar palsy (BP) are characterised by dysarthria, dysphagia and dysphoria.

PBP is caused by bilateral upper motor neurone lesions in the corticobulbar pathway leading to dysfunction of IX, X, and XII cranial nerves leading to spasticity of the tongue and a pathologically brisk jaw jerk. Rapid alternating movements of the tongue become difficult. Bilateral lesions of the corticospinal tracts are associated with upper motor neurone signs in the limbs. There is a characteristic gait with short steps, 'marche a petit pas'. The syndrome commonly involves emotional lability and/or dementia. The facial appearance is mask-like. Choking attacks are distressing and frequent.

BP involves lower motor neurone signs of the same cranial nerves resulting in weakness, wasting, and fasciculation of the tongue. The dysarthria has a nasal quality and the weakness of the muscles involved in swallowing leads to nasal regurgitation and aspiration. Lower motor neurone signs may occur in the limbs.

Poor voluntary movement has been described in both conditions.

AO'H

10.

(a) Axis I   – major clinical syndrome
     Axis II   – developmental and personality disorder
     Axis III – physical disorders
     Axis IV   – severity of psychological stressor
     Axis V   – highest level of adaptive functioning in past year.

(b) Family studies – show clustering in families
     Twin studies – show higher concordance in monozygotic twins (42%)
          than in dizygotic twins (9%)
     Adoption studies – show that adopted away offspring of parents with
          schizophrenia still have an increased risk of schizophrenia.

(c) Higher relapse rates in schizophrenic patients who had families which
     showed high expressed emotion (EE), who spent over 35 hours each
     week in the high EE environment and who were not taking
     neuroleptics. High EE includes overinvolvement and critical
     comments during interview.

PDM

11.

(a)   Hypothyroidism
        Cushing's syndrome
        Addison's disease
        Hyperparathyroidism.

(b)   Reserpine depletes presynaptic vesicles of amines and may precipitate
        depression.
        Tricyclics and MAOIs increase the amount of amines in the synaptic
        cleft and improve depression.
        Amphetamines can induce euphoria and cause increased levels of
        synaptic amine by release of amines from presynaptic vesicles.

(c)   Foods high in tyramine: cheese, broad bean pods, red wine, pickled
        herring, hung game, meat extracts, liver, flavoured textured vegetable
        protein, alcoholic or non-alcoholic beers.

                                                                        PDM

12.

Risk factors:
        young male
        recent hospital discharge
        depression
        social isolation
        good previous education
        hopelessness
        chronic relapsing illness

Predictors of poor outcome:
        early onset
        no precipitants
        insidious onset
        family history of schizophrenia
        low IQ
        no affective symptomatology
        social isolation
        poor pre-morbid personality
        low social class
        hebephrenic or simple schizophrenia
        presence of neurological soft signs
        assaultative behaviour   PDM

13.

(a) 'Safe limits' are up to 21 units weekly for men and up to 14 units weekly for women, provided there are drink-free days and the whole amount is not taken in a single bout.

'Hazardous levels' are 21–49 units weekly for men and 14–35 units weekly for women.

'Dangerous levels' are above these limits.

(b) Have you ever felt that you should Cut down your drinking?
Have you ever felt Annoyed at people who have criticised your drinking?
Have you ever felt Guilty about your drinking?
Have you ever had an 'Eye opener' (a drink on waking) to steady your nerves?

Two positive replies are said to indicate problem drinking.

PDM

14.

Freud's psychoanalytic theory presupposes that our actions are determined by inner forces and impulses which operate at an unconscious level. Freud described two opposing instincts: the life instinct (eros) and the death instinct (thanatos). Energy associated with either instinct can build up and discharge either inwardly or outwardly. Aggression can be the outward expression of energy associated with the death instinct. By contrast social learning theory rejects the notion of an innate drive and claims that aggressive behaviour is a learned response; learned through observation or imitation (vicarious learning). Re-inforcement increases the likelihood that the behaviour would be learned. An aversive experience leads to emotional arousal. This arousal may lead to aggression. The increased general arousal may reduce cognitive appraisal of the immediate environment and the anticipated consequences of actions. The interaction between the individual and his environment is emphasised. Aggression may occur as a coping mechanism. This contrasts with the unconscious destructive urges in Freudian theory.

AO'H

15.

(a) Pragmatism stresses the purposive nature of cognitions. The key to the meanings of concepts or beliefs is seen in terms of their practical consequences. Language understanding in conversation requires an understanding of pragmatics, equivalent to our general world-knowledge.

(b) Analogic communication is concerned with all non-verbal communication e.g. tone of voice, facial expression, body posture and all forms of physical contact. Analogic messages are also communicated through appearance (such as clothing and hairstyle), music, painting and poetry. Digital communication involves the communication of facts in written or spoken form.

(c) Relationships can have symmetrical and/or complementary interactions. A symmetrical interaction is one where both individuals are on an equal footing. They suggest equality. Complementary interactions suggest a hierarchy with the two individuals occupying different positions relative to one another. An example of this might be a dyadic relationship where one partner is dominant and the other submissive.

(d) Semantics refers to the meaning of words, the relationship between words and symbols and the overall meaning of language. The meaning of a word can be equated with what it refers to in the real world, although this approach runs into difficulties with abstract words like 'justice' or 'morality'. Another approach is to equate the meaning of a word with the mental image it summons up, but this too runs into problems with respect to abstract words. More complex semantic theories look at words as bundles of semantic features or associations. The theory of prototypes looks at how we classify words and concepts: we have a prototypical idea of what a bird is. Some birds may fit this prototype better than others. A robin may be closer to an individual's prototype of a bird than an ostrich. The concept of bird and birds then is held together by a family resemblance structure.

AO'H

16.

(a) *Four from:*
  Tardive dyskinesia
  Rabbit syndrome
  Parkinsonism
  Acute dystonia
  Akathisia
  Tardive dystonia
  Tardive akathisia

(b) Parkinsonism develops early in the treatment phase (a few days to a few weeks) and may remit spontaneously despite continuing neuroleptic treatment. Early management may involve reassurance for mild symptoms which may remit, but pharmacological management using anticholinergic drugs such as procyclidine can be justified. Reduction of the antipsychotic drug dose may be beneficial if a reduction is feasible. A substitution of another antipsychotic with a reduced side-effect profile is sometimes necessary. Amongst phenothiazines, those with a piperazine side-chain show more extreme extrapyramidal effects than those with aliphatic or piperidine side-effects.

Acute dystonia may occur rapidly after the initial administration of a phenothiazine (24–48 hours from start). It appears to be related to individual susceptibility as well as to the dose and type of antipsychotic. Treatment is by parenteral administration of an anticholinergic such as procyclidine 10 mg i.v. This may need to be repeated as necessary before oral medication begins to work, but maximum dose should not be exceeded. Response is dramatic. Occurrence of a previous dystonic reaction is one of the few indications for prophylactic use of anticholinergic drugs with neuroleptics.

Tardive dyskinesia (TD) is considered to be a long-term complication of neuroleptic treatment. It is potentially irreversible even if the antipsychotic drug is discontinued. There is no effective treatment. Management involves using the lowest possible doses of antipsychotic medication for the shortest period of time. Neuroleptic treatment should be withdrawn if possible, although this may be unrealistic. In the majority of situations the TD is mild and no other treatment is necessary. In some cases a change to a different class of neuroleptic may be helpful. Addition of noradrenergic antagonists, e.g. propranolol, or the addition of GABA-affecting drugs like benzodiazepines may be useful on a short-term basis. Vitamin E and calcium-channel blockers have been used in individual patients with some success. The role of anticholinergic drugs in the causation of tardive dyskinesia is unclear.

AO'H

17.

1. Ensure patient is in a safe environment, with use of the Mental Health Act for compulsory admission to hospital if patient is unwilling to be admitted voluntarily.

2. Appropriate and judicious use of medication to relieve distress e.g. major tranquilisers or benzodiazepines (use of the latter with care in view of possible disinhibiting effects).

3. Clearly stated (and written) guidelines for management for all staff involved.

4. Ensure no means of self-harm are available to the patient (knives, ropes, plastic bags, caches of tablets).

5. Adequate ward supervision: 1 to 1 nursing observation. Prevent patient leaving ward alone whilst suicidal ideation persists, with recourse to Mental Health Act if not already invoked.

6. Thorough medical review and regular reviews of mental state and suicidal ideation and plans. Current suicidal ideation to be communicated to key members of staff.

7. Ensure long-term management plans are made in terms of early ECT for major depressive disorder. If patient consent is not forthcoming, a second opinion will be required.

8. Nurse on ground floor if possible.

9. Avoid frequent changes of nursing staff.

10. Identify a carer who will allow the patient time to relieve his distress in a compassionate, containing environment.

18.

(a) Reliability involves the extent to which a research instrument gives consistent results if used on the same sample more than once under the same conditions.

  – split-half reliability looks at the correlation between a randomly chosen half of the questions and the other half.

  – test–retest reliability looks at the correlation between test scores when the test is administered to the same group on different occasions.

  – inter-rater reliability is measured when different observers have rated the same series of patients and the ratings are compared.

  – alternate-form reliability is where two tests are administered, the second being a modified form of the first.

(b) *Five from:*
Definition: defining the exact type/source of patients taken into the study (inclusion/exclusion criteria), defining the form of therapy to be used: may involve use of manual, and level of expertise of therapists.

Measurement: measuring change in therapy during process and outcome, defining criteria to be used, ratings by therapists, patients, or independent observers. Should measurement be during, at end, and/or at follow-up of therapy.

Controls: waiting-list, or alternative type of therapy, age/sex-matched

Sample size: problems in finding and enrolling enough patients in all groups (treatment and control), finding enough therapists and maintaining their involvement to completion. Magnitude of placebo response can be quite high necessitating large groups e.g. 100 plus. Initial numbers may need to be larger because of attrition in various groups. Study design affects power.

Generalisation: is the group used in the research representative of the general clinical population? Is the therapy a recognised form, or can it be taught and replicated by others?

Missing data: through drop-outs from groups or courses of therapy.

Ethical considerations: disclosures during therapy, confidentiality, worsening clinical state and involvement of outside agencies. Is a waiting list or placebo group ethical in moderate depression, bearing in mind the possible delays before 'recognised' treatment is used.

Confounding factors: use of anxiolytics, alcohol, antidepressants and other drugs, secondary therapists being drawn in.

BG

19.

(a)   temporal lobe epilepsy
transient ischaemic attacks
post-traumatic confusion
encephalitic illness
migraine

(b)   depression
vitamin B_{12} deficiency
hypothyroidism
cerebral tumour
general paresis

(c)   cerebral atrophy (with ventricular dilatation, sulcal shrinkage, cerebellar atrophy)
perforation of septum pellucidum
loss of neurones in cerebral cortex
neurofibrillary degeneration
gliosis of mid-brain

BG

20.

Six different types of intracranial tumour:

Gliomas
    astrocytoma
    glioblastoma multiforme
    medulloblastoma
    oligodendroglioma

Meningiomas

Blood vessel tumours
    angioblastomas
    angiomas

Tumours of the pituitary and third ventricle
    craniopharyngiomas
    chromophobe adenomas
    prolactinomas
    colloid cyst of third ventricle

Acoustic neuroma

Metastatic tumours (lung, breast, stomach, prostate, thyroid)

(a) Frontal lobe
    pre-frontal:
        headache (later papilloedema and vomiting)
        progressive dementia
        generalised convulsions
        expressive dysphasia (if Broca's area involved)
        grasp reflex unilaterally
        facial/tongue weakness
        anosmia
    pre-central:
        focal convulsions: Jacksonian attacks
        motor weakness: contralaterally
        apraxia/weakness of face and tongue on opposite side
        reflex abnormalities

(b) Temporal lobe
        temporal lobe epillepsy
        generalised fits
        crossed upper quadrantic hemianopia
        tinnitus
        auditory hallucinations
        aphasia in left-sided lesions – difficulty naming objects
        jargon speech
        associated with III nerve palsy

(c) Corpus callosum
        apathy
        drowsiness
        memory defect
        depression

anxiety
epileptiform convulsions
if expands into frontal lobes may have grasp reflex
apraxia
high protein content of CSF

BG

Further reading

Abbot RJ, Loizou LA (1986) Neuroleptic malignant syndrome. Br J Psychiatr, 148, 47-51.

Addonizio G, Susman VL, Roth SD (1986) Symptoms of neuroleptic malignant syndrome in 82 consecutive patients. Am J Psychiatr, 143, 1587-90.

Casey D (1991) Neuroleptic drug-induced extrapyramidal syndrome and tardive dyskinesia. Schizophrenia Res, 4, 109-20.

Chadwick (1989) Medical Neurology. London, Churchill Livingstone.

Delay J, Deniker P (1968) Drug-induced extrapyramidal syndromes. In: Handbook of Clinical Neurology, vol. 6. Diseases of the Basal Ganglia. New York, Elsevier.

Graham P, Rutter M (1985) Adolescent disorders. In: Rutter, Hersov (eds), Child and Adolescent Psychiatry. London, Blackwell.

Jones KL, Smith DW, Ulleland CN, Streissguth AP (1973) Patterns of malformation in offspring of alcoholic women. Lancet, 1, 1267.

Rogers D (1992) Neuropsychiatry of movement disorders. Curr Opin Psychiatr, 5, 84-7.

Rossett HL (1980) A clinical perspective of the foetal alcohol syndrome. Alcoholism Clin Exp Res, 4, 119.

Royal College of Psychiatrists (1986) Alcohol: our favourite drug: a report of a special committee. London, Tavistock.

Stephens JH, Astrup C, Mangrum JC (1966) Prognostic factors in recovered and deteriorating schizophrenics. Am J Psychiatr, 122, 1116.

Stillings NA, et al. (1987) Cognitive Science. London, MIT Press.

Vaillant GE (1964) Prospective prediction of schizophrenic remission. Arch Gen Psychiatr, 11, 509.

Vaughn C, Leff JP (1976) The influence of family life and social factors on the course of psychiatric illness. Br J Psychiatr, 129, 125-37.

Weinstein MR (1980) Lithium treatment of women during pregnancy and in the post-delivery period. In: Johnson N (ed), Handbook of Lithium Therapy. Lancaster, MTP Press.

Yalom ID (1975) The theory and practice of group psychotherapy. New York, Basic Books.

The Essay Paper

APPROACH

Follow the instructions for labelling your answer paper with your name and choice of essay carefully. Work out where you will plan your answers. Evaluate each of the six alternatives very carefully, and work out how you might approach each one. There will inevitably at least one option you would never dream of attempting, but there should be two or three titles that you could reasonably address.

Of those two or three you could best do, work out a brief plan of what you could confidently write about in each. Pick the one of these that you could write most about, and which you feel most enthusiastic about and flesh out your brief plan.

Write legible, brief sentences. Make each point as succinctly as you can, and elaborate only when you are adding to (rather than re-iterating) what you have already said. Make references to solid research where possible (but do not be tempted to grandiosity by trying to quote volume numbers, pages etc.), and explain its relevance to the point you are trying to make.

Your essay should follow a logical line of thought, paragraph by paragraph. If it does not, then it will lose relevance to the original question and you will be wasting time writing unwanted material.

The essay papers are designed to provoke some discussion and debate in your answer, rather than trigger a regurgitation of facts. The clarity of your argument, your ability to evaluate evidence and your ability to synthesise a longer piece of work are being tested as well as your knowledge base. The subjects of the essays may focus on some point of debate in recent research or psychiatric services.

Use the example paper that follows by trying to work out a plan for each of the six questions.

MRCPsych Part II
One-and-a-half hours
1 essay out of 6

Write an essay on ONE of the following six topics:

1. You are asked to provide independent advice for a group of purchasers as to what psychiatric services they should purchase for a population of 100,000.

2. What are the applications of the cognitive therapies? How do they compare with pharmacological therapies in terms of efficacy and compliance?

3. "We will soon be able to attribute the causes of mental illness to specific genes as a result of gene mapping research programmes." Discuss the truth of this statement with additional consideration of recent research into the genetics of schizophrenia and bipolar affective disorder and the ethical implications for psychiatry in the future.

4. "Affective disorders are usually reactions to loss events." Discuss with reference to research on life-events and personality.

5. "Childhood bereavement and parental loss and repeated separations from attachment figures . . . are associated with increased rates of depression in childhood and later life, and therapeutic intervention with children facing or experiencing loss improves their mental health and functioning." This statement appeared in an editorial by Dr Dora Black in the *British Medical Journal* (Mental Health Services for Children, 305, 971-2).

   Discuss, with evidence, the assertions in this quote and explain what evidence there is that childhood psychological distress is manifest in adult life?

6. What are the objectives for psychiatric services outlined in the 1992 White Paper *The Health of the Nation*? How might these be realistically achieved? What other measures could be employed to evaluate community mental health and mental health services?

BG

Patient Management Problems

GENERAL APPROACH

The patient management problem oral examination lasts for half-an-hour, during which two examiners pose a variety of problems for you to answer. An average of four may be presented to you. To do well would be to satisfy the examiners on as many PMPs as possible. Past examinees, though, have passed by answering as few as two PMPs in considerable depth.

The key to the PMP is to appear competent and confident, although not overly so. The examiners must be left with the impression that you would be safe as a consultant. Wild guesses, extraordinary body language, and blatant attempts to show-off esoteric knowledge will ruin this impression. As much as anything, examiners are interested in whether you have a strategy for analysing problems which can be generalised in your clinical life.

Listen carefully to the problem outlined by the first examiner. The problem should not be over-long or over-detailed. What detail there is in the question is usually vital to the diagnosis or management so try to use all the detail in your reply. Address routine matters first – in assessing patients there are steps which you might take for granted, but, unless you mention them, the examiner will have no idea whether you know them or not. The difficulty here is in balancing the need to explain yourself against the distinct possibility of boring the examiners. You alone can judge this in the exam setting. Sometimes examiners will move candidates on to the area they are particularly interested in if they are satisfied that your general approach is correct. Another strategy for the candidate is to 'go for the jugular' and address the most important part of the PMP first. If the PMP sounds like a 'barn-door' case of neuropsychiatric complications of systemic lupus erythematosus you could say this immediately, but almost in the same breath you must emphasise that you would still go through the usual careful assessment procedure that you always do. This up-front strategy avoids the impression that you are waffling around, talking about assessment, when you haven't a clue as to what the diagnosis might be.

There is no ideal way to answer PMPs that will work with all PMPs for all candidates and all examiners. PMPs can be in diverse subspecialities – mental handicap, child psychiatry, forensic psychiatry and others. Your main asset will be the ability to think 'on your feet'. In terms of preparation you should begin practising your skills for the PMP exam as early as possible. Ward rounds and case conferences are good training grounds for voicing your thoughts on patient management. You may also find peer groups useful in practising PMP exam technique. A trio of exam candidates can act in turn as candidates and examiners, having each thought up several PMP-style questions.

During the exam itself the PMPs you are working on may evolve. After you have discussed assessment, the examiners may feed back investigations such as EEG or CT scan reports. You may have to moderate your initial impressions. After you have formed a working differential diagnosis, the examiners might ask you for your ideal management. Remember that management may include pharmacological, family, social, and individual psychological interventions in a variety of settings (day hospital, outpatients, day centres, community clinics and inpatients). You must be confident to talk about the management of easy and resistant cases of depression and schizophrenia. An increasing emphasis may be placed in the future on knowledge of psychological techniques. How is a behavioural program structured in detail? What goes into a cognitive-behavioural diary in managing bulimia? If you don't know something in the exam, try to apply basic principles, but don't present dangerous wild guesses, say, about the exact dosage regime of phenelzine.

You will have gained the impression from the above that the PMP exam is very interactive. Both examiners will ask you PMPs and both will have different styles which you will need to adapt to, although their approach is standardised as far as is possible by initial training as examiners and the sometime presence of Royal College observers who may take the form of a 'silent' fourth person in the room.

Some patient management problems will require you to refer to legal procedures used in compulsory admissions for assessment and treatment. The College is aware that, depending on where exam candidates live and work, their familiarity with the English and Welsh Mental Health Act may vary. If you are most familiar with Irish or Scottish legislation, you should make this clear to the examiners in the PMPs and the Clinical test. This will avoid any misunderstanding on the examiners' part. In the following PMPs and responses, we have referred to the 1983 Mental Health Act in use in England and Wales.

The exam may focus on particular difficulties in management, such as how to manage resistant depression or schizophrenia. These and other problems in management which you should be fully conversant with are usefully discussed in *Dilemmas and Difficulties in the Management of Psychiatric Patients* (Hawton K, Cowen P (1990) Oxford, Oxford University Press).

BG

PATIENT MANAGEMENT PROBLEMS: A Personal View and Some Hints on How to Play the Game

It would be ideal if your natural ability as a psychiatrist and clinical acumen was all that was tested in the PMP part of the exam, but in the real world this is not the case. While sound clinical judgement should be a basic essential requirement of any candidate who has reached the Part II exam, this often becomes one's least preoccupation when facing the examiners.

The first aspect to take into account is *how the examiners see you.* You could show professorial knowledge to your peers, or be praised ad nauseam by the consultants you work with, but none of that counts on the day. All that matters is the 30 minutes the examiners see of you. Before turning to consider how you should set about answering their questions, let us first pay attention to the first impressions they will form of you as you walk in the room and sit facing them across the table. First impressions should not be that important, but examiners are human (believe it or not!) so first impressions count for a great deal. Also, if you dress and adopt a posture that looks as if you mean business, then your attitude when answering the questions will tend to follow the same path.

Your appearance should look as if you will be a competent consultant psychiatrist (which, after all, is what the exam is all about). This generally means wearing a dark suit (men) or something equivalent (women). In my (female) opinion, women should wear a skirt (not too short) and preferably have any long hair neatly tied back. Having said that, the overriding rule should be that you feel comfortable and reasonably natural in whatever you wear: it is no good dressing up to look like someone you are not, as this is likely to make you feel uneasy while talking, and perhaps come across as unconfident to the examiners (more of that later).

Your posture is also crucial. Think about how you will walk into the room and sit down! That may sound daft, but if your head is lifted high and you walk in boldly, perhaps immediately making eye-contact with one of the examiners, and then sit down in a calm manner, that will all be to your benefit. Think about your body language while you are sitting. We are all so used to making judgements about patients by the way they sit in a chair, yet are surprised if other psychiatrists do the same to us.

Sit fully on the chair; sitting on the edge will make you look anxious and hence unconfident. You may say that the examiners should realise that any candidate would naturally be feeling anxious, so it should not matter. Unfortunately it does matter. Firstly, the examiners are themselves quite anxious (they may not have met each other before; one of them may not have examined before) so the last thing they want is for someone to sit there and make them feel worse! Secondly, any impression that you are feeling unconfident almost invariably leads to the erroneous impression that you are also incompetent. If there is one thing that you have to convince the examiners of, it is that you are basically a competent and safe psychiatrist. So you should try at all costs not to display your natural anxiety.

Think of yourself going into the exam as a salesperson, selling yourself instead of computers, but using the same principles. Make as much eye contact as possible with the examiner who is questioning you (without staring). If you really cannot bear looking straight at the whites of the examiner's eyes, practice looking at a spot on the wall at the examiner's eye level, behind him: this will give the impression that you are looking at him when you are not! Also, don't forget to smile. This will prevent you looking unsure while you are thinking of your answers.

Many salespeople practice their technique either in front of a mirror or in front of a video camera. You must do the same. I used to cringe at the thought of seeing myself on a video: but it really is an exercise worth putting yourself through. I suggest that you find a friend or colleague who can act as a mock examiner (preferably someone doing the exam at the same time as you, so that you can both be inflicted with equal torture by each other). Lay the room out similarly to an exam room: the examiner should sit behind a table, and your chair be directly facing him. Place the video camera behind the examiner, focused directly onto the candidate; that way the picture will truly be of you as the examiners see you. Then go through a mock viva. It does not really matter what questions are asked; all that is required is that they put you under some pressure (without deteriorating to an argument!) so that your demeanour and attitude when under stress can be looked at. I was unpleasantly surprised by how much I fidgeted when nervous: mannerisms, which inevitably make people seem anxious, should be reduced to an absolute minimum.

Answering the questions posed also requires some practice. There is a convention that your answer should follow the same route as your formulation in the clinical exam would. So you always start with assessment (have a schema in your head of what you run through in a history, mental state, physical examination so that you do not miss anything out); investigation; management. Bear in mind also the triad of 'physical, psychological and social'; and remember that histories can be obtained from individual patients, but also from close relatives, whole families, other agencies (like social workers) or institutions (like employers or schools), as well as from previous case notes!

In medicine there is often an exception to an 'always'. I would say that the exception to your answer 'always' beginning with assessment is if there is some information of overriding importance that you want to make sure you have time to let the examiner know you know. This generally arises in situations where life is somehow in danger. For example, if given a description of someone who is or could be suicidal, I would begin with: "My prime concern here is for the patient's safety, and I am concerned that she may be a suicide risk, but I would begin by assessing . . ." This shows the examiners you are thinking safely, but allows you also to then go through the conventional pattern of answering, and you can return to discuss the suicidal intent in more detail later on.

The exception described above should not be abused. There is often a temptation, especially when adrenaline is pumping through your veins, to envisage some rare small-print syndrome that might fit the description given by the examiners. By all means keep that whim at the back of your mind, to earn extra points after you have given your textbook reply, but stop yourself from mentioning it before anything else. Common things occur commonly, and the examiners will be perfectly satisfied if you have a good working knowledge of the main syndromes.

If you are asked a question you do not understand, do not waste time: just ask the examiner to repeat it: the chances are the other examiner had not understood it either. Do not be thrown by questions about the obscure: everybody has their own ceiling, and it may just be that they are testing you to see how well you can perform.

When the examiner goes on to the next PMP, try to put the previous one completely out of your head. You have to earn points on each one, so try to begin with a completely clean slate each time.

CPR

Below are a selection of PMPs by different authors. They are followed by sample answers. The responses are not meant as ideal or 'model' answers, only as examples of possible ways of answering the PMP. You might like to try to formulate your own answers before reading our examples. There is some representation of how interactive the PMPs can be, because, in our examples, the examiners do come back with supplementary questions. In practice there is likely to be more interaction.

1. The Asthmatic

The medical team ask you to see a 21-year-old girl who is currently on a medical ward for a severe attack of asthma. She may soon need ventilation. The patient is refusing this and wants to take her own discharge. Her asthma is usually controlled with inhalers but she stopped these herself. Her asthma is complicated by a small pneumothorax. She has seen a psychiatrist in the past. She has a history of deliberate self-harm dating from the age of 14.

On interview, she is breathless, and has successfully detached herself from a drip of hydrocortisone. She has also been treated with nebulised bronchodilators. She gives a history of low mood with an onset six weeks before the asthma attack, and describes current tearfulness, poor appetite, and early morning wakening. She has ideas of worthlessness, delusions of guilt and second-person auditory hallucinations telling her that she should kill herself. The patient is disorientated in time, but not in place or person.

How would you respond to the physicians' request for help?

This is a complex case which would need careful assessment, but also seems to merit a swift response. On what I have been told there are grounds for using the Mental Health Act to detain this patient. Firstly there is evidence of a mental disorder (low mood preceding the attacks, and current psychotic features) and secondly, the patient is at risk of harming herself because of self-hate and second-person auditory hallucinations telling her to kill herself. It may also be that her decision to reject treatment is based on a desire to harm herself. On this basis there would be a case for not allowing her to discharge herself and using a section. Since she is an inpatient, Section 5.2 *could* be applied by the RMO, but Section 2 proceedings might be preferable. This would allow treatment of her mental disorder, but treatment for any physical illness would fall under Common Law. Her mental disorder affects her ability to give valid consent at this time (given that there are psychotic features and disorientation). After a Section has been invoked, joint evaluation and treatment by medical and psychiatric teams would be necessary. Their aims would be to improve her respiratory function and assess and treat her mental disorder.

There is a history of low mood preceding the asthma attack which might indicate an underlying depressive illness, although she is quite young to develop this. I would take a careful drug history. For instance, had she been on steroids for any great length of time? Steroids could have produced her psychotic state. Her disorientation could be due to hypoxia. As her respiratory function improved, her disorientation might improve, and so might some of her psychotic symptoms.

At this point the examiner intervenes to give further information. Some second-person auditory hallucinations had preceded the asthma attack, and continued after her asthma attack was over. She was not on steroids before this admission.

In which case a major depressive episode seems more likely, with a hypoxic disorientation overlying this. The patient or an informant could give a clear history of the depressive illness.

So, given that she is now on the Mental Health Act Section 2, how would you treat her?

This would have to be in conjunction with the physicians, but I would be keen to gain rapid control of her depressive illness. ECT might be the treatment of choice, if there were no respiratory contraindications. Her respiratory function and recent pneumothorax might concern the anaesthetist. An antidepressant like fluoxetine or sertraline might be an alternative. If there were associated behavioural disturbance, I would recommend a neuroleptic with less sedative properties like haloperidol.

Have you any thoughts about her personality, given her history of deliberate self-harm? She has cut her wrists in the past and taken overdoses as a teenager.

My assessment would also include her account and an informant's account of her pre-morbid personality. I would consider the possibility that there was a personality disorder. Her asthma attack (precipitated by a failure to take treatment) might have been a deliberate act of self-harm too. However, given the immediate presentation, I would be careful to assess and treat any depressive illness.

Further reading:

Jourdan JB, Glickman L (1991) Reasons for requests for evaluation of competency in a municipal general hospital. Psychosomatics, 32, 413-16.

Kopelman LM (1990) On the evaluative nature of competency and capacity judgements. Int J Law Psychiatr, 13, 309-29.

Wear AN, Brahams D (1991) To treat or not to treat: the legal, ethical and therapeutic implications of treatment refusal. J Med Ethics, 17, 131-5.

BG

2. A Panic Attack

A casualty SHO asks you to see a forty-five-year-old lady. She has just had a 'panic attack' and fainted while shopping in the centre of town. She talks to you of her anxieties about her daughter's impending wedding (she had been in town to buy a hat for the wedding). You notice that she smells of alcohol, which she spontaneously explains. A shopkeeper had given her some brandy to revive her. However, on physical examination you notice that she has palmar erythema, a tremor and a pulse rate of 104 beats per minute.
How would you propose to further assess and manage her?

The smell of alcohol and the palmar erythema would make me suspicious that this lady abuses alcohol. I would review her alcohol history particularly carefully, seeking confirmation from a relative or other informant. The informant might be able to give valuable information about the panic attack, which I am unclear about. Was this really a panic attack induced by general anxieties about a forthcoming wedding? Or was it perhaps a symptom of agoraphobia, or an attack of syncope, or an alcohol withdrawal fit? The history would clarify some of these issues, particularly about the form of the actual attack itself. It would be important to exclude medical causes such as a rhythm disturbance.

An examiner intervenes to inform the candidate that there was no irregularity in the pulse, but that there was tachycardia.

Yes, so I would be interested not only in the history and physical examination but also in some investigations. Specifically, I would request an ECG, but also a full blood count (in case of anaemia), a urea and electrolytes (for dehydration) and serum glucose (to exclude hyper- or hypoglycaemia). A thyroid function test would be important to exclude hyperthyroidism which might be the cause of any anxiety and tachycardia. Liver function tests including a gamma-GT and the MCV on her full blood count might exclude prolonged alcohol abuse.

Let us suppose that all the initial casualty investigations come back normal. Perhaps her tachycardia resolves when she has talked to you a bit more about her difficulties at home. You have been careful enough to get the medium-term investigations like LFTs and TFTs done and, obviously, are awaiting their results.

Well then I would be interested in her past psychiatric history. Were there any episodes of agoraphobia in the past? Has her GP given her any treatment for anxiety? Perhaps with benzodiazepines? And particularly ask about her family relationships. Perhaps the panic is to do with her daughter leaving home, some structural change in the family. I would try to get an opportunity to talk to the husband . . .

The examiner interrupts because he is satisfied with this line of enquiry and has only a few points to cover before closing down. He acknowledges the role that psychological factors may play in the presentation, but asks what pharmacological alternatives there would be to psychotherapeutic measures.

Particularly if there was an element of general low mood, an antidepressant such as imipramine might help. Imipramine has been reported to be of value in panic disorders. MAOIs have been used for agoraphobia and panic disorder, but there might be difficulties using irreversible MAOIs in someone with an alcohol problem. So I would consider an MAOI such as moclobemide which does not have such severe dietary restrictions as the older irreversible MAOIs. Propranolol *could* have a role if there were a more generalised anxiety, but you would have to check whether there was any predisposition to asthma. Benzodiazepines would certainly reduce the anxiety, but would not be of any medium- or long-term benefit.

BG

3. The School Non-attender

You are sent a referral by a school medical officer. He refers you a 13-year old girl who has barely attended school in the last half term (it is now half way through the autumn term). She has always been a good attender until now. Her school work has also suffered. She was a most able pupil. Now she has slipped to being near the bottom of the class.

How would you set about managing this problem?

This case requires outpatient assessment, but does need a swift response as her schoolwork has apparently suffered quite markedly. The assessment will involve seeing the girl herself and making a family assessment. I would get information (if parents allow) from the school and any other interested parties such as the Educational Welfare Officer.

A very important area to cover in the history of the presenting problem is whether or not this is school refusal or truancy. Is she staying at home with her parents' knowledge? Or is she pretending to them that she is attending, and either not turning up at all, or leaving very early in the school day? Does she truant in a group with friends, or (more worryingly) on her own? If she is truanting, what does she do during the day? (Drug abuse, glue-sniffing or shop-lifting are particular worries.)

A clear indication of the duration of the problem is required – did it really start after the end of the summer holidays? What were the

147

antecedents? Is she currently attending school? What statutory moves have been made to get her back to school? An indication of whether the school has a sympathetic attitude towards her case or not is useful.

The examiner explains further that this is a case of truancy. Occasionally she truants with other girls (who were not previously her friends). However, much of the time she never turns up at school, and appears to go into town on her own. She denies any substance abuse and simply says she wanders round the shops all day. The school has been so worried about her behaving out of character that no legal moves have yet been made.

Her mother says that she became more moody, and more difficult to talk to, since her periods began. Her periods started just after the end of the previous summer term.

What does this make you think of?

Of prime importance here is this girl's probable very low mood. I would elicit any suicidal ideas or plans. Evidence we already have for a depression would be her truanting alone, deteriorating school performance, and a change in behaviour at home as well.

My next concern would be the cause of this depression. The timing of the problems just after the menarche is vital. There are several ways in which the onset of periods can be disruptive for a teenager. The impact may depend upon what the girl expected beforehand and how her family (and especially mother) reacted to her menarche. Her peers may have teased her about it. There is also the possibility of sexual abuse and its consequences.

CPR

4. The Soiler

A GP asks you to see a six-year-old boy who soils himself at least once every day. How would you set about this?

I would obtain a thorough history. It would be worth finding out from the GP what investigations and treatment(s) have been attempted, and over what length of time. The whole family should be seen, to take a history, including duration and onset of the problem, also the precise circumstances around current episodes of soiling. It is very important to determine whether the boy has been adequately toilet trained. A clear past history, including his position in the family, and current family and school circumstances, is required. This assessment may need several meetings with the family. Teachers' opinions and reports should be sought.

The pattern of the soiling itself will need examining. Is aggression a main motive behind it? Are there associated behaviours such as smearing? Is he constipated (suggesting a more retentive pattern)? Eliciting the precise antecedents and consequences of specific incidents of soiling can be very informative.

The examiner elaborates the history by explaining that the soiling only occurs at home, never at school, and follows a retentive pattern. He was clean and dry from the age of two until six months ago. Furthermore, his parents separated over a year ago, and are getting a divorce. The boy is the elder of two children, his sister being four years old and showing no problems at all.
What else do you want to know?

The parents' separation and divorce seem linked in time to the start of the symptoms. I would ask about the state of the parents' marriage beforehand, also about current difficulties. I would like to know precisely what the boy has been told about what is going on.

The father is a long-distance lorry driver who used to be away in Europe for several days at a time. He left his wife a year ago for another woman (who was expecting a baby by him and which was born six months ago). Both his original children stayed with their mother. The mother had been very upset by the break-up. Since then, her husband had started requesting access, but even before that they were frequently rowing about this.
How would you now manage this case?

The access dispute is the major perpetuating factor here, so resolution of this between the parents will be a major help in relieving the stress borne by the boy. Conciliation work may be required for this.

The divorce may not have been adequately explained to the six year old: so it should be ensured that the situation is clearly and unambiguously explained to him. Ideally, both parents should do this together: but this may not be practicable, so they may need to do this independently.

Addressing these two issues will be tackling the probable causes of the encopresis. However his soiling may have taken on the nature of a habit, so that, even when these factors have been removed, behavioural techniques may also be required, including star charts, consistent reactions to soiling, and positive rewards (specific to the child himself) for remaining clean. A hierarchy of achievable targets should be created. Also, the boy may be so severely constipated at presentation as to require 'clearing out' with laxatives or even, in exceptional circumstances, an enema before the behavioural treatment programme can be embarked on.

CPR

5. The Addict

A 26-year-old woman is referred to your drug dependency clinic by a consultant obstetrician. She is 12 weeks pregnant, wants to keep the baby, and has told her that she is a heroin addict. How would you proceed?

In order to manage this patient, I would want more information from the patient and an informant. I would want to confirm that she is in fact a heroin addict. I would want to know more about her drug use, her general circumstances, her motivation to stop taking drugs and her knowledge of the health risks she is taking. I would want to be able to discuss other details with the obstetrician.

The first thing is to get a full history of her drug habit. I would want to know which substances, including alcohol, she takes, how much of them, and for how long she has been using them. I would need to know whether she injects now or in the past, and whether she has ever shared needles. Is her habit funded out of legitimate income or crime? If she is a prostitute or has shared needles, there is a risk of hepatitis and HIV. I would ask about any periods of abstinence from drugs or drink and how they were achieved. Has she ever had treatment or help for substance misuse in the past?

I would need to know about her general social circumstances: housing, employment and support from family, friends and/or partner. I would look for any evidence of mental illness, and predisposing, precipitating and maintaining factors for her heroin addiction.

Physical examination would be important for evidence of drug use such as weight loss, constricted pupils, and intravenous puncture marks, venous thromboses, abscesses, sinuses – looking in the groins, neck and legs as well as the arms. Breast veins are sometimes used in late pregnancy. I would also look for any signs of septicaemia or endocarditis. I would take a full blood count, liver function tests, hepatitis and syphilis screening, and might consider offering HIV tests if appropriate. Such testing would need to be after appropriate counselling. Urine samples should be sent on more than one clinic attendance to confirm the presence of opiates (bearing in mind any prescribed medication she might be taking as some of these may interact with testing).

I would assess her motivation to stop taking heroin. Ultimately, she may want to stop completely or become stabilised on oral methadone.

I would, with her permission, interview an informant, perhaps a partner, to check the information I have been given and to enlist their support in her treatment. Discussion of the management with her GP and obstetrician would help.

Since she is in the early stages of pregnancy, she should be stabilised on methadone rather than withdrawing her completely, because of the risk of spontaneous abortion. The methadone could be prescribed mg for mg with heroin, but the starting dose would have to be calculated with great care since the purity of street heroin varies enormously. The first goal would therefore be for her to stop using street heroin, and to stop injecting and any relevant criminal activity.

I mentioned the risks of stopping opiates completely in the first trimester and, for the same reason, reducing her methadone in the first trimester would not be advisable. Reducing her methadone in the last trimester might induce premature labour. It *might* be possible though to reduce her methadone gradually in the middle trimester.

What about any legal implications of her seeking help from you?

At the first appointment, I would have to tell her that I was legally obliged to notify her name to the Chief Medical Officer because there is a register of addicts.

And what about the baby? Would there be any short-term or long-term consequences?

If the patient does not stop taking drugs during pregnancy, the baby is likely to be born drug dependent and would need very careful management of withdrawal symptoms. In the long-term, there would be implications if the mother is HIV-positive and if the baby is born HIV-positive. The child would then be at risk in terms of cognitive decline in infancy and HIV-dementia. If there is no HIV infection then the child may still be at risk of conduct or other childhood psychological disorders if their environment is chaotic. There is evidence to suggest that, if the mother continues to use heroin in the years to come, then her child is more likely to use heroin too.

Further reading:

Glynn TJ (1981) From family to peer: a review of transitions of influence among drug using youth. J Youth Adol. 10, 363-83.

Hepburn M (1993) Drug use in pregnancy. Br J Hosp Med, 49, 1.

Nurco DN, Hanlon TE, Kinlock TW (1991) Recent research on the relationship between illicit drug use and crime. Behav Sci Law, 9, 221-42.

Smart RG, Fejer D (1972) Relationships between parental and adolescent drug use. In: Keup W (ed), Drug Abuse: Current Concepts and Research. Illinois, Charles C. Thomas.

PDM

6. The Arsonist

How would you assess a patient referred because of setting a fire?

I would take a detailed history of the fire-setting to see if the act was pre-meditated or impulsive, carried out alone or with others and whether it was part of a pattern of previous fire-setting behaviour. I would be interested in the factors that motivated the patient – such as covering up some other crime, insurance fraud, revenge, political motivation, sexual gratification or re-inforcement, delusional ideation, suicidal ideation, or the wish to appear a hero, perhaps by calling the fire brigade.

I would take a full psychiatric history and make a thorough mental state assessment, looking for evidence of mental illness, mental retardation, alcohol dependence or personality disorder, all of which have been linked to fire-setting behaviour.

An informant would be essential for a corroborative history.

Three groups of arsonist have been described: motivated arsonists – ones motivated by political or financial reward; pathological arsonists suffering from mental illness such as depression, mania, schizophrenia, mental retardation or alcoholism; and a third group who derive sexual enjoyment from fire-setting or who derive better self-esteem from heroic acts at 'their' fire. A key point of the assessment would be of the patient's dangerousness.

What would make you think they were likely to repeat the fire-setting behaviour in the future?

A history of previous arson, mental retardation and poor insight, dissocial personality disorder, social isolation, and fire-setting re-inforced by sexual arousal and masturbation, or re-inforced by tension relief.

Further reading:

Gelder M, Gath D, Mayou R (1989) Oxford Textbook of Psychiatry, 2nd Edn. Oxford, Oxford Medical Publications, 880-9.

Kolko DJ, Kadzin AE (1991) Motives of childhood firesetters: firesetting characteristics and psychological correlates. J Child Psychol Psychiatr, 32, 535-50.

PDM

Clinical Examination Advice

INTRODUCTION

Both parts of the MRCPsych examination incorporate clinical exams. In the first part the emphasis is on psychopathology and differential diagnosis. In the second part the candidate will have to demonstrate clinical skills and an ability to make a good differential diagnosis, but will also be expected to be fully conversant with management issues and prognosis.

The reason for failure of the clinical examination cannot be laid at the patient's or examiner's door. The fault can only lie in the candidate's preparation, presentation and discussion of the case.

To increase the chance of passing the clinical examination, the candidate must have considerable experience in presenting patients in an examination-like setting, and be confident enough to overcome any anxiety.

There are three rules: rehearsal, rehearsal and rehearsal.

PREPARATION

In the context of a busy service, the candidate must make time for a formal rehearsal at least once a week for two or three months before the examination. The prerequisites of a good session are:

1. The patient is new to the candidate.

2. The session is devoted to examination rehearsal.

3. The time spent both with the patient and the examiner is as near to the examination format as it can be.

4. The examiner asks probing questions.

5. The examiner is truthful and constructive in feedback.

6. The session should be formalised to the extent that it may reproduce a mild degree of anxiety for the candidate.

The ideal session is very difficult to come by in real life. However approximations can be achieved through:

Formal presentations in ward rounds.

Peer syndicates being arranged locally in which potential candidates present cases to each other.

Video presentations.

GENERAL POINTS

The clinical examination and patient management problems are usually held at the same centre on the same day. The day is long enough and stressful enough without the difficulty of getting all the way from home to the centre by car or train that day. Arrive the day before and stay overnight in a nearby hotel. Stay in comfort and treat yourself well! Eat a hearty breakfast! Dress comfortably so as to look confident, but also dress smartly and soberly. Dark, conservative colours are the order of the day. Try to look 'consultoid', and be comfortable in that attire.

CONSTRUCTING THE PRESENTATION

Most medical cases are formally presented by working through a list of headings. Psychiatric cases are no exception. The potential candidate will be familiar with the order of assessment and presentation, given here in Table 1 (for the sake of brevity, I have cut out detail).

Table 1: The Order of Assessment

---

reason for referral	personality
complaints	mental state
present illness	appearance and behaviour
family history	talk
personal history	mood
development	thought
medical/psychiatric	abnormal experiences
forensic	insight
alcohol/drugs	cognitive examination

From the information elicited under each of these headings, the candidate constructs a differential diagnosis, or this is what is supposed to happen. In fact, usually somewhere half way through the 'present complaint', the psychiatrist has generated preliminary diagnoses. During the rest of the interview, many of the questions will be asked in order to substantiate this.

Consequently, when presenting the case, the examinee should present it so that data under each of the relevant headings substantiates the differential diagnosis that he/she comes out with at the end. During the presentation of the case, it is of course important to emphasise these cardinal features.

The case may not be clear cut in that there is data substantiating more than one diagnosis. This must not be seen as a problem but as an interesting area of debate to present to the examiners. In this particular situation, the evidence supporting one diagnosis is balanced against the evidence supporting the other. As is recognised by most classification systems, the patient may have more than one diagnosis.

When there is little or ambivalent clinical evidence, making it difficult to produce a firm differential diagnosis, the candidate must make it clear how further information is to be collected within the management plan of the case.

In presenting the case to the examiner, the candidate builds up evidence supporting the diagnosis with which he/she concludes the presentation.

CONSTRUCTING THE MANAGEMENT PLAN

The management plan is more the preserve of the Part II examination rather than the Part I, which focuses on psychopathology and differential diagnosis. Part I candidates should therefore read the following for interest's sake. The initial part of the management concerns the recruitment of further data to substantiate the diagnosis. The management plan should be divided into two:

	Data collection	*Treatment*
Early management: Physical		
Psychological		
Social		

	Data collection	*Treatment*
Later management: Physical		
Psychological		
Social		

Using headings of this nature, the candidate is less likely to omit important components.

THE PROGNOSIS

As with management, prognosis is usually explored in the Part Two examination only. Any statements you make must be justifiable. The clear-cut case is a relative rarity and to say the prognosis is good, poor or bad without qualification will almost certainly lead to further questioning by the examiner.

The examinee may get away with general terms that do not commit, providing a framework for further discussion within the examination; terms such as 'guarded' or 'cautiously optimistic'. These phrases mean relatively little on their own and might lead to further examination. The best approach is to consider the prognosis in terms of immediate (concerning the particular episode) and longer term. In this context the examinee can present the immediate prognosis as good but draw attention to the poorer long term prognosis. An example of such a case is a patient presenting with depression who has a history of recurrence or strong personality traits that might make the individual prone to relapse.

EXAMINATION TIME

Time spent with the patient: This is the critical part of the clinical. How the candidate spends this time determines to a great extent whether the examination is passed or failed.

The objectives are:
    to examine the patient
    to establish a differential diagnosis
    to construct a management plan
    to work out the prognosis
    to rehearse the presentation

When the examinee first enters the room where the patient is waiting the anxiety will be high but reduces quite quickly. Some examinees will 'freeze' initially. One way of overcoming this initial anxiety is to:

Introduce oneself to the patient, explain the exam set-up and that, because time is against you, you may have to cut them short. Try to get the patient 'on your side' as much as possible.

Take three or four minutes to write out the headings of the

presentation (as above), well spaced on a side of paper (a crib sheet). This can be used as a guide during the history taking, it may also be of use later in the examination. This exercise gives the candidate a sense of mastery and will focus thinking, taking the edge off any anxiety. The examinee can now get on with taking the history, taking notes as normal. This should be completed with ten or fifteen minutes to spare at the end for thinking time.

Write down the differential diagnoses. Five broad headings can be considered:

psychoses (schizophrenias etc.)
organic
neuroses (including eating disorders)
personality
affective disorders.

It is often useful to have a short classification list in mind as one of the common fears of examinees is that 'something' has been missed. Such a list offers a simple clinical 'sieve'.

The next stage is to write down one word cues covering the main salient features of the case under each of the headings on the crib sheet (Table 2). This will allow presentation of the case to the examiners without reading from notes word for word.

The last five to ten minutes of the time left to the candidate can be best spent in presenting the case. This can be done by asking the patient to sit quietly for a few minutes. As the candidate you might turn to face the wall and present the case to yourself in a muttered voice. It is quite important to go through this verbatim as, in doing so, you will not fall into the trap of taking short cuts and will therefore have to think the case through. More importantly, you will be going into the examination having already presented the case.

It may also be worth thinking about likely items the examiners will ask you to demonstrate when you interview the patient in their presence. Key factors of psychopathology may be chosen by the examiners. You could alert the patient beforehand to the kind of questions that you may be asking later. Remember the patient will be just as anxious as you about performing in front of the examiners.

Table 2: An example crib sheet

Crib sheet summary:

Patient's ID: Mr Pretend, 42 years, engineer, not worked for 6 months, married, in hospital two weeks (referred by GP).

History of present complaint:
  3 months ago: saw road traffic accident
  Cries most days
  Early morning wakening
  Diurnal variation
  Irritable
  Sex drive down
  Appetite loss
  Lack of energy
  Frightened of being away from wife

Family history: Mother: long-term 'nerve' trouble.

Personal history:
  Father died when patient was six
  Disturbed elder brother: violent, drugs, theft
  Difficult schooling: Mum kept him at home
  Job after school
  Lived with mum until married at thirty-five
  Married
  Teetotal
  No previous psychiatric history

Personality: Dependent, low confidence, prone to withdrawal when under stress

MSE:
  Appearance and behaviour: weepy, poor eye contact, stooped, wrings hands, dishevelled
  Talk: quiet voice, poor spontaneity, mono-syllabic
  Mood: sad, low self-esteem
  Thought: hopeless, pessimistic, self-depreciative, non-delusional, no suicidal thoughts or plans
  Percept. NAD
  Cognition: some psychomotor retardation

Differential:
Depression
Dependent traits in personality (NB: early loss)

Management:
Immediate: data collection
Physical: examination, blood tests
Psychiatric: observe for endogenous features, sleep and appetite monitoring, assign key nurse to explore psychology (NB watch for suicidal ideation)
Social: SW and examine domestic and work dynamic. Explore premorbid personality
Treatment:
Physical: commence antidepressant
Psychiatric: key worker to build relationship
Social: depends on social assessment
Longer term:
Physical: treat conditions found
Psychiatric: management of medication; duration and compliance
Psychosocial: psychotherapy

Prognosis:
Short term: good
Long term: dependent personality will make him vulnerable to future stress. Possible risk of recurrence

---

PRESENTING THE CASE

The presentation should begin with a very brief introduction to the case, giving the name, age, occupation and where and with whom he/she lives, and the duration and nature (in-patient/out-patient) of current contact with the psychiatric service. This assessment should fill ten minutes or so.

Having just spent an hour with the case and having already rehearsed the presentation, the examinee should be confident enough to use the crib sheet. This allows eye contact with the examiners and gets the examinee out of the temptation of reading notes.

The examinee must demonstrate that he/she is confident and organised. Keep good eye contact with the examiners. Reply to questions using first person.

When psychopathology is referred to in the presentation, a verbatim example is often asked for, so be prepared. It is important that the examinee has the courage of conviction concerning the presence or absence of psychopathology, stating firmly whether the patient is or is not exhibiting the phenomenon.

Do not include diagnoses within the differential that cannot be specifically justified. A great mistake is to be over-inclusive and then to be made a fool of when one cannot explain why it was included except 'safety' reasons.

Avoid the term 'organic' in differential diagnoses. If the patient is thought to be suffering from an illness of this nature, then try to be specific and present evidence as to why this diagnosis had been thought of.

When giving the mental state examination, make sure that the appearance of the case is not, for example, just described as 'depressed' but 'as a person with poor eye contact, brimming of the eyes, hunched shoulders, wringing of the hands'. Spend a little time on the appearance and behaviour, describe important features of the personal presentation that contribute towards the differential diagnosis. Such a description is quite impressive.

When the patient is interviewed in front of the examiners be careful to show your awareness of the discomfort that the patient might be experiencing. Turn your chair sideways to the examiner, facing the patient and not the examiners. This makes the interview into a two-way interchange, looks impressive to the examiner and makes the situation much more controllable.

If asked a question by the examiner that is ambiguous or needs clarification, do not hesitate to ask for clarification.

Read and be aware of the guidelines issued by the Royal College on the time generally allocated to items such as 'presentation' and 'patient interview' (Table 3).

Table 3: Guide to time spent with examiners in Part II Clinical

Assessment	10 minutes (approx)
Interview with patient	5 minutes (approx)
Management)	10 minutes
Prognosis)	(approx)
Further discussion	5 minutes (approx)

With practice the candidate will become adept at interviewing the patient, arranging information and will have enough time for a brief rehearsal. The essence of passing the clinical examination is to go into it confident and organised. To achieve this it is essential to control anxiety, this is done by extensive rehearsal in the context of a well established routine which is fail safe.

KW